Arthritis

Made Simple!

MALIN PRUPAS, MD, FACP

Arthritis Made Simple!

Interior illustrations by Maureen Burdock.

Published by Wheatmark®
610 East Delano Street, Suite 104
Tucson, Arizona 85705 U.S.A.
www.wheatmark.com

ISBN-13: 978-1-58736-619-2
ISBN-10: 1-58736-619-3
Library of Congress Control Number: 2006925634

This book is dedicated to my patients. Regardless of their pain and suffering as a consequence of their arthritis, they continue to go about their daily activities and lives. They encourage me to measure success in inches, rather than miles. As they turn their cheek and keep their head high, they encourage scientists and doctors to continue to look for further treatments and interventions that will benefit mankind.

Contents

Acknowledgments

My patients taught me about arthritis and the fascinating manifestations of more than one hundred different illnesses. How phenomenal that the same disease looks so different in each individual person. Books taught me the facts, my professors taught me the skills, and my wife and family made my work passion all possible.

Introduction

The withdrawal of successful painkillers like Vioxx (rofecoxib) and Bextra (valdecoxib) from the market has added to the confusion about the treatment of arthritis. Even so, there are several new therapies on the horizon. There is a lack of practical information available about arthritis and its treatment for health professionals and patients. This book is intended to be a simple explanation of a difficult subject.

Arthritis is a chronic disease. Arthritis affects everyone in the family. Millions of Americans have some form of arthritis, and one in three families is touched by it. As the American population gets older, musculoskeletal problems will become more important and frequent. The social and economical impact will be significant. Health care providers are preparing for this now. In recognition of the importance of promoting bone health and preventing fractures, the president of the United States declared 2002–2011 as the Decade of the Bone and Joint. Thus, the nation has committed resources to accelerate progress in a variety of areas related to the musculoskeletal system, including bone disease and arthritis.

Autoimmunity

The immune system normally makes proteins (antibodies) that protect the body against viruses, bacteria, and other foreign materials (antigens). However, in an autoimmune disorder, such as lupus, the immune system loses its ability to tell the difference between foreign cells and its own cells and tissues (self). As a result, the immune system incorrectly makes antibodies directed against itself. These autoantibodies react with the self-antigens to form immune complexes. The immune complexes deposit in various tissues and create inflammation, injury to tissues, and pain. More than 70 percent of people with systemic lupus have these antibodies deposited in different parts of the body. Several types of arthritis are characterized by specific autoantibodies and the immune complexes they form. These antibody markers are not foolproof, but serve as markers distinguishing diseases and the activity of disease.

This immunological mechanism is the body's defense and is characterized by redness, warmth, swelling, and pain at the site of inflammation. The inflammation at a wound site will bring more blood, including specialized white cells to defend against infection, to the area. Healing begins as the inflammation subsides. Inflammation at the cellular level may not be visible, as is a sore on the skin. Chronic inflammation may be deleterious to good health. The inflammatory response of the body is measured by the C-reactive protein (CRP) in the blood. The inflammation measured by the CRP may contribute to the progression of heart disease. Reduction of inflammation in heart patients has been shown to reduce the progression of atherosclerosis linked to heart attacks and death.

Inflammation may be the link between increased risk of cardiovascular disease and early death in rheumatoid arthritis. Researchers have known that patients with rheumatoid arthritis have a higher mortality rate from heart disease than those individuals without rheumatoid arthritis. The exact mechanism—and whether the CRP measures the actual mechanism that causes plaques in the arteries or is just a sign of it—is un-

known. While researchers unravel this complex issue, it is important that physicians pay more attention to the cardiovascular status of patients with arthritis.

Rheumatology

Rheumatology is an internal medicine subspecialty providing care to persons with arthritis and related conditions. Rheumatism is a generic term describing all forms of arthritis. Rheumatic illnesses are primarily diseases of the immune system and other disorders that cause pain and inflammation of the joints, muscles, and bones. Osteoarthritis, rheumatoid arthritis, gout, systemic lupus erythematosis, bursitis, and osteoporosis represent some of the many forms of arthritis. Arthritis involves much more than just the joints. When arthritis affects multiple other organ systems of the body, it becomes a systemic illness. Arthritis patients obtain their care from rheumatologists, primary care physicians, and other allied health professionals.

Timely consultation with a rheumatologist can help ensure a positive outcome after a prompt and accurate diagnosis and initiation of appropriate therapy. Coordinated management by the primary care physician, specialist, and therapist is desirable. A rheumatologist can often diagnose and treat arthritis less expensively than doctors not specifically trained in arthritis management.

CHAPTER ONE

Identifying Arthritis

The pain of arthritis is forever. Arthritis may be one symptom of a more serious disease. A swollen, red, painful, and hot joint is inflamed. Arthritis literally means joint inflammation. Unfortunately, most types of arthritis are chronic and last a lifetime. The diagnosis and early management of arthritis is imperative. Early treatment makes a difference. The most common types of arthritis include rheumatoid arthritis, osteoporosis, systemic lupus erythematosis, fibromyalgia, gout, seronegative spondyloarthropathies, scleroderma, and osteoarthritis.

Major Warning Signs of Arthritis
◊   swelling in one or more joints
◊   early morning stiffness for one hour
◊   continual or recurring pain in one joint
◊   difficulty moving a joint
◊   warmth or redness of a joint
◊   nodules under the skin
◊   joint pain with fever, weakness, weight loss, or rash

Rheumatoid arthritis is a symmetrical inflammatory type of arthritis. For example, if one knee is swollen, the other knee may be swollen, perhaps not at the same time. Rheumatoid arthritis is a polyarthritis (more than five joints). This is in contrast to monoarthritis, or one swollen joint. Rheumatoid arthritis primarily affects young and middle-aged women between twenty and forty-five years of age. Men and children are also susceptible to rheumatoid arthritis. The small joints of the hands are especially involved, but so are the larger joints like the hips, knees, ankles, shoulders, and elbows. Other organ involvement includes the skin, eyes, heart, muscles, lungs, bones, and nerves. There is a genetic predisposition, although the details are still not totally understood. The cause is actually unknown. More than one family member may be affected. The joint inflammation tends to be characterized by exacerbations (flares) or periods of inactivity (remissions). The course of the arthritis is characterized by periods of peaks and valleys that last days, weeks, or months. Rarely, spontaneous remissions occur and the arthritis burns itself out. Of one hundred consecutive individuals put in the hospital and followed closely for an extended period at the time of the onset of rheumatoid arthritis, a small number will have a short-lived illness that will resolve without intervention, a small number will have a terribly active form of the disease that destroys the joints quickly, and the majority of individuals will have a persistent ongoing illness. These individuals develop increasing complications of rheumatoid arthritis, loss of function, radiographic destruction, and disability over many months or years.

Osteoporosis is a condition in which bone mass, bone density, and bone strength decrease. This results in an increased susceptibility to bone fracture. After menopause, levels of the female hormone estrogen decrease and bone loss increases. This puts older women at risk for fragility fractures (a fall and fracture from standing height). The loss of estrogen diminishes the beneficial effects on bone. If estrogen replacement therapy is not given during this time, a rapid loss of bone occurs. Recent discovery of the effects of estrogen replacement therapy in postmenopausal women, such as increased heart rate, stroke, or breast cancer, has influenced many women to discontinue estrogen replacement therapy. Stopping estrogen later in life has the same effects on the bone as naturally occurring menopause. Unless other interventions are instituted after menopause, bone loss occurs later in life. Bone loss occurs more often in Caucasian and Asian populations. Osteoporosis occurs in association with other diseases and with the use of some medications, especially corticosteroids. Symptoms do not occur until there is a fracture, commonly of the hip, wrist, or spine. Spinal fractures result in loss of height or dowager's hump. Bone density measurements done by dual energy x-ray absorptiometry are a useful and simple way to look for the risk of fracture and measure treatment effectiveness. Screening dual energy x-ray absorptiometry scans are now readily available.

Systemic lupus erythematosis is a form of arthritis that is not uncommon and actually occurs more often than well-publicized illnesses like multiple sclerosis or leukemia. The antinuclear antibody is found in almost all individuals with systemic lupus erythematosis.

Systemic lupus erythematosis patients are usually women of childbearing ages. However, the very young, the elderly, and men also develop systemic lupus erythematosis. About five hundred thousand Americans between the ages of fifteen and forty have systemic lupus erythematosis. A small number of people develop systemic lupus erythematosis after taking medications that induce autoimmunity. Think of the illness as a long railroad track. At one end of the track are those individuals with serious problems, including involvement of the brain, nerves, or kidney. At the other end of the track are those with less serious disease like achy joints (arthralgias), fatigue, or skin rash. Immune complexes are deposited anywhere in the body. The location of the deposited immune complexes determines the signs and symptoms of the disease. Nonspecific symptoms of systemic lupus erythematosis include photosensitive rashes, hair loss, alternating color changes of the fingers, joint pain without swelling, mouth ulcers, fatigue, and seizures.

Fibromyalgia is known as fibrositis, myofascial pain syndrome, soft tissue rheumatism, or nonarticular rheumatism. The syndrome includes trigger point pain well mapped out on the body's surface, poor sleeping habits, and mild depression. These events occur in a vicious cycle associated with marked fatigue. Symptoms snowball, get worse, and send the patient in a downhill spiral, bouncing from one doctor to another doctor to another without any clear diagnosis or treatment plan. Many fibromyalgia patients see multiple physicians without an answer for their symptoms and have surgery trying to achieve pain relief. The longer the duration of symptoms, the worse the prognosis. People often benefit from antidepressant medication at bedtime (to improve sleep and mood), learning about their illness, and support groups. Alternative health care is actively sought out.

Gout is a crystal-induced arthritis. Gout is one of the oldest forms of arthritis. Inflammation of the joint is precipitated by the deposition of crystals of uric acid. The crystals precipitate a powerful and painful response by the body. All gout patients have high levels of uric acid at some time or another, although not necessarily at the time of an acute attack. The serum level of uric acid should not be used to make the diagnosis. The majority of patients are middle-aged men or postmenopausal women. The first attack usually occurs in the big toe, although gout can affect many joints at once and mimic other forms of arthritis. Attacks begin infrequently, but eventually occur more often. Treatment includes anti-inflammatory medications, given during the acute attack. The treatment of the elevated uric acid levels includes drug therapy, either to promote excretion of uric acid in the urine (uricosuric drugs) or to inhibit the formation of uric acid in the serum (hypouricemic drugs). Drugs that lower the serum uric acid should not be started during an attack. Decreasing the uric acid level rapidly may precipitate, prolong, or worsen an acute attack of gout. Special diets are not necessary. Patients with gout tend to be overweight and hypertensive. Gout patients are the only rheumatology patients that come to the arthritis clinic wearing slippers, cutout shoes, or sneakers, or using crutches, because they are so uncomfortable. The pain is excruciating.

Seronegative spondyloarthropathy is more common in men than women. More than 90 percent of patients have the genetic marker HLA-B27. About 6 percent of the normal population has the same genetic marker without arthritis. The forms of arthritis in this group include ankylosing spondylitis, psoriatic arthritis, Reiter's syndrome, and the arthritis associated with inflammatory bowel disease. Ankylosing means rigid or stiff, *spondyl* refers to the spine, and *itis* means inflammation. The inflammation results in the vertebral bodies of the spine growing together slowly, usually over many years. Other organ systems outside the musculoskeletal system are also involved.

Scleroderma occurs more commonly in women than men, but not exclusively. Another term for scleroderma is progressive systemic sclerosis. Subtypes include localized scleroderma (morphia) or eosinophylic fasciitis. Not unique to progressive systemic sclerosis is a characteristic color change of the fingers (Raynaud's phenomenon). Other characteristics include calcifications just under the skin (calcinosis), diminished esophageal motility, dilated small vessels under the skin (telangiectasia), and tightening of the skin at the fingers (sclerodactyly). Scleroderma literally means hard skin. Progressive systemic sclerosis is potentially life threatening due to damage that occurs to internal organs after excessive accumulation of the protein collagen. Lung or kidney involvement is a poor prognostic indicator and encourages aggressive management of complications.

Osteoarthritis, or degenerative joint disease, is the most common form of arthritis. By age sixty, most individuals have some evidence of osteoarthritis or wear-and-tear arthritis. Weight-bearing joints are prone to involvement, including the hip, knee, or spine. Modern surgical techniques have made replacement of hip and knee joints common, successful, and safe in every community hospital. Anti-inflammatory medications and mild analgesics provide symptomatic relief but do not change the course of the arthritis. Joint trauma results in osteoarthritis later in life. Whether overuse plays a role in causality remains to be proven. Involvement of the distal interphalangeal (DIP) joint at the end joint of the finger (Heberden's node) and the proximal interphalangeal (PIP) joint or middle joint of the finger (Bouchard's node) affect a unique genetic subset of individuals with osteoarthritis, usually women. Diffuse idiopathic skeletal hyperostosis (DISH) is a severe form of degenerative joint disease affecting the spine.

CHAPTER TWO

Rheumatoid Arthritis

One percent of the adult American population, or greater than two million Americans, has rheumatoid arthritis (RA). RA is more common in women as compared to men, in a ratio of about three to one. Rheumatoid arthritis frequently affects people in their most productive years, between the ages of twenty and forty-five with the peak between thirty-five and forty-five. Disability because of RA results in major economic losses.

Most people with RA develop a detectable rheumatoid factor (RF) in the blood. Those with a negative RF or early disease are difficult to identify but have a better prognosis. Recently, identification of early RA with a detectable anti-cyclic citrullinated peptide antibody (anti-CCP) has been helpful in those individuals without a detectable RF. The fluctuating course characterized by peaks (bad times) and valleys (good times) of activity makes it difficult to clearly define the arthritis early.

A small number of individuals with new onset RA will have a short-lived illness, which will resolve after a few months. Future research may indicate that these people did not have RA or that there are several forms of the arthritis. Most individuals will have a lifetime of disease with joint destruction, the development of deformity, and disability. A small number of patients will have a severely destructive form of the disease (arthritis mutilans) and never have any periods of inactivity. Studies reveal an increase in death rates among these patients, as compared to the general population, especially in those individuals with severe progressive joint involvement.

Those with multiple joint involvement or polyarticular disease, persistent swelling, a detectable RF, a detectable anti-CCP, or evidence of bone destruction or erosions discernible by x-rays have a greater probability of more severe disease than those who do not have these symptoms. Joint damage and destruction occur early during the course of the disease and necessitate an early diagnosis and treatment directed by a rheumatologist.

Disease Process of Rheumatoid Arthritis

The typical joint has a capsule that surrounds the entire joint space. The capsule attaches to the bone above the cartilage. This leaves an exposed area of bare bone. One or two cell layers of synovial cells form a microscopic synovium and line the inside surface of the capsule. In RA, the synovial cells multiply, grow, and a thickened pannus formation develops. Inflammatory cells migrate into the synovium and create synovitis. The synovium is aggressive and invades the exposed area of bare bone, just above the normal cartilage. Proliferative synovium becomes obvious to the naked eye. Once the synovium invades the bone, radiographic erosions (breaks in the cortex of bone) develop and the arthritis destroys the joint. The joint is severely changed and deformed.

Erosions

Periarticular bone erosions near the joint surface are characteristic of RA as compared to the destruction caused by other types of arthritis. Thickened

Typical Joint

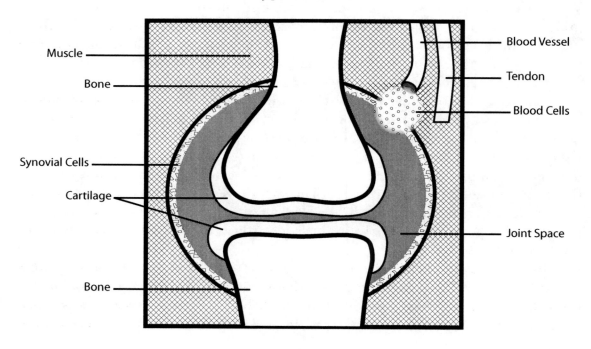

synovium or pannus allows fluid, inflammatory cells, destructive enzymes, and chemical mediators of inflammation or cytokines to enter the joint space. The cartilage loss appears on the x-ray as uniform narrowing of the joint space. Thickened or "turned on" synovium is evidence of active disease. The area around the joint becomes vascular. A biopsy of the synovium reveals nonspecific inflammation.

The x-ray changes of RA are different from the changes of osteoarthritis (OA) and help distinguish between the two different illnesses. In OA, the joint is narrowed irregularly, not uniformly as in RA. In OA, the bones develop spurs. The x-ray is usually distinctly different from the inflammatory changes of RA. The x-ray of RA is characterized early by periarticular demineralization on both sides of the joint space, later by uniform narrowing of the joint space, and finally by erosions around the joint as a result of the synovial pannus invading bare areas of bone not protected with cartilage. The final outcome is total destruction of the joint and misalignment.

The prognosis of RA is determined by the history of the course and onset of the arthritis, evidence on examination of persistent pain and swelling, laboratory findings, x-ray changes, extra-articular manifestations, and current level of patient function. Poor prognosis deserves aggressive treatment.

Extra-articular RA involvement outside the musculoskeletal system significantly affects prognosis and the severity of disease and treatment. The most common extra-articular manifestations include anemia, rheumatoid nodules, a detectable rheumatoid factor, rheumatoid lung disease, and vasculitis of the skin. Pulmonary involvement includes interstitial lung disease, fibrosis, or scarring of the lung, pulmonary nodules that resemble cancer, and pleurisy or fluid in the chest cavity. Vasculitis of the skin results in painful skin lesions or ulceration of the skin.

Determining the Prognosis of Rheumatoid Arthritis
◊ early age at onset
◊ positive rheumatoid factor (RF)
◊ positive anti-CCP
◊ nodules or vasculitis
◊ extra-articular manifestations
◊ x-ray changes
◊ early disability

Upper Extremity

Rheumatoid arthritis affects the hands and feet, rather than the central joints of the body like the spine as does OA. Early in the disease, the hand appears normal, but as time passes, physical changes define the course of the arthritis. The metacarpalphalangeal joints (MCPs) sublux downward and the

The Hand and Wrist

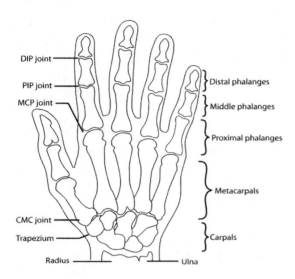

DIP joint
PIP joint
MCP joint

Distal phalanges
Middle phalanges
Proximal phalanges

Metacarpals

CMC joint
Trapezium

Carpals

Radius — Ulna

fingers develop ulnar deviation. Subluxation of the joint of the thumb results in a Z-shaped deformity, or "90-90" thumb, and makes it difficult for the patient to grasp anything by pinching it. Synovitis of the wrist results in loss of motion. Grip strength is diminished. Occasionally, the fourth or fifth extensor tendons of the fingers rupture and the fingers can no longer be extended or held out straight.

Rheumatoid nodules occur at the elbow in conjunction with swelling or accumulation of fluid at the elbow bursa. Fixed elbow flexion contractures are common. It is difficult to see swelling at the shoulder. Keeping the shoulder motionless because of pain results in loss of motion, a frozen shoulder, and adhesive capsulitis. Regaining lost shoulder motion is difficult. Loss of motion occurs quickly in any joint not moved regularly, or held motionless, during the day.

Lower Extremity

Quadriceps muscle wasting of the thigh occurs quickly after the onset of synovitis of the knee. Joint fluid accumulates at the back of the knee and forms a cyst. This creates a fullness or tightness of the knee. A ball and valve mechanism forms a one-way valve that keeps sending more and more joint fluid to the popliteal space of the knee. This creates a tight popliteal cyst (Baker's cyst). If the cyst gets too full, the cyst ruptures and creates a sudden onset of pain and swelling down the calf, mimicking deep venous thrombosis. Treating the synovitis prevents accumulation of the inflammatory fluid sent to the popliteal space and the resulting symptoms. Popliteal cysts should not require surgical intervention.

At the foot, the toes go in the opposite direction of the fingers. This puts extra pressure on the metatarsal heads while weight bearing. The pain created is called metatarsalgia. Calluses form over the pressure areas. Cocked-up toes rub on shoes, cause skin irritation, and require meticulous foot care. Skin ulcers occur, and they can get infected. The forefoot widens, and bunions occur at the first big toe. A widened forefoot makes it important to find proper fitting footware. Subtalar joint involvement below the ankle prevents normal inversion and eversion of the foot.

As the disease progresses, hip involvement becomes more likely. Early hip pain is localized to the groin or even radiates to the knee. Later, hip arthritis results in more widespread pain and pain at night. Limping is common. Use of a cane on the nonpainful side is helpful and shifts the weight to the other side. If there is arthritis of the hands and wrists, a cane is difficult to use.

Other Joints

Although the temporal mandibular joint (TMJ) is similar to other joints and affected by RA, symptoms are unusual. Inflammation of the joints controlling the vocal cords causes hoarseness or sore throat. Except for the upper cervical spine, most areas of the spine are spared by the involvement of RA. Subluxation of the first two cervical vertebrae is common and initially won't cause symptoms. Cervical subluxation is frequent in those individuals with more severe disease. A modest separation is significant and often requires surgery. At surgery, the two vertebrae are fused to prevent pressure on the cervical spinal cord (myelopathy).

The cause of RA is uncertain. Although not entirely understood, on occasion more than one family member has RA. Genes that influence the immune system are inherited and create a susceptibility to the disease. Unknown factors cause the disease in those individuals with a genetically susceptible immune system. There are some researchers who believe the unknown factor is an infectious agent, which triggers the immune system to react abnormally. Pregnancy is associated with remissions during the third trimester with subsequent exacerbation in the postpartum period. The effect of pregnancy on RA suggests hormonal factors play a role in disease activity.

Criteria to Identify Rheumatoid Arthritis
◊ morning stiffness around the joints lasting one hour
◊ arthritis and swelling of three or more joints simultaneously
◊ arthritis of the hand joints
◊ symmetrical arthritis
◊ rheumatoid nodules
◊ detectable rheumatoid factor
◊ x-ray changes typical of rheumatoid arthritis

Polypharmacy of Rheumatoid Arthritis

Concurrent multiple drug therapy is the basis of the drug treatment of RA and other autoimmune illnesses. The treatment of RA is rapidly changing and deserves special mention in comparison to the drug treatment of other diseases. Drug therapy slows the course of RA, as compared to its effect on OA. Rheumatoid arthritis treatment was once based on a series of building blocks that slowly tapered and diminished in size to form a pyramid. At the base were safer modalities like acetaminophen, aspirin, and NSAIDs. As the pyramid got higher, the selections were fewer in number, but they were more potent and had greater potential for side effects. The treatment of RA is now considered polypharmacy and the pyramid has been inverted. Several drugs in combination at the same time are used early in the disease course. This requires meticulous attention to possible drug interaction. The rheumatologist possesses the special skills and experience in the use of these different medications. Perhaps more than in any other field, the evaluation and treatment of RA is a true exercise in the art of medicine and good judgment.

Experience has proven that the treatment of RA must be aggressive. Potent medicines must be used early in the disease course and in those individuals with poor prognostic signs. Studies show that patients with active disease and other predictors of a poor prognosis develop joint damage or erosions of bones near the joint early, within two years of onset of the disease. Poor prognostic factors are determined by physical exam, the laboratory, or x-ray. Most rheumatologists favor early aggressive treatment

of patients with evidence of active inflammation. Intervention should occur within the first few months that the diagnosis is definitely established. Unfortunately, there is no magical pill in the treatment of any form of arthritis.

Some of the oldest methods of arthritis treatment are now being questioned. Older drug therapies are falling by the wayside because of important biotechnical discoveries able to target directly specific areas of inflammation or disease. Scientific studies done with medication for the treatment of RA must be interpreted carefully for both efficacy and risk. Efficacy includes the benefits and risks include the side effects. If a medication does have side effects, it is hoped that any new problem is not as severe as the disease itself. If the side effects are severe, then the medicine should be discontinued or kept to a minimum.

Polypharmacy of Rheumatoid Arthritis
◊ miscellaneous medications
◊ analgesics
◊ anti-inflammatory agents
◊ disease modifying anti-rheumatic drugs

The drugs used in the management of RA are divided into four different categories: miscellaneous medications, analgesics for pain, anti-inflammatory agents, and disease-modifying antirheumatic drugs (DMARDs). It is important to know something about each group and how the medications work in concert.

Miscellaneous Medications

Miscellaneous medications include several different drugs, but are not limited to estrogen replacement therapy for postmenopausal women, antibiotics for infections, antihypertensives for the treatment of high blood pressure, cholesterol lowering agents, or perhaps something simpler like an over-the-counter vitamin or calcium tablets. Drug interactions are carefully monitored. Patients with RA or other autoimmune disease are at special risk for stomach ulcers, infection, kidney problems, and osteoporosis. Other problems should not be ignored. Since most patients are women, there may be special needs around the time of menopause including calcium and vitamin supplementation. The years of potential childbearing require effective contraception. Drug regimens need modification during pregnancy or breast-feeding. Many acid-blocking drugs like nizatidine (Axid), famotidine (Pepcid), cimetidine (Tagamet), or ranitidine (Zantac) are available over-the-counter. More potent acid-blocking medications like rabeprazole (Aciphex), pantoprazole (Protonix), omeprazole (Prilosec) or lansoprazole (Prevacid) esomeprazole (Nexium) require a prescription. Misoprostol (Cy-

totec) replenishes prostaglandins, which play a key role in inflammation but a protective role for the stomach lining in the body's defense against its own gastric acid.

Analgesics

Analgesics treat pain and include opioids (narcotics). Opioids require cautious and judicious use. Pain relievers mask pain without actually changing the course of arthritis. While treating a chronic incurable disease like RA with only narcotic analgesics, there is always the possibility of the patient developing dependence or even addiction to pain medications. Narcotics need not be avoided, but should be kept to the lowest possible dose that does the job. Opioids impair emptying of the stomach and bowel mobility, which leads to constipation.

There are some narcotic medications that have a greater potential for abuse and should probably be avoided if possible, including oxycodone with aspirin (Percodan) or oxycodone and acetaminophen (Percocet), pentazocine (Talwin), meperidine (Demerol), or hydromorphone (Dilaudid). The use of these medications must be individualized to the needs of the patient. Oral oxycodone has ten times the analgesic effect of codeine. The active metabolite of meperidine can lead to CNS excitability.

In some cases, individuals in need

of total joint replacement are unable to get surgery done immediately. Pain relief is still essential and these individuals require narcotics. Long-acting narcotics like morphine (Oxycontin) or fentanyl transdermal patches (Duragesic) provide many hours of continuous safe pain relief throughout the day. Dependency must be watched for in these patients. The rule of thumb about narcotics is more is not always better. Fentanyl has a rapid onset of effect.

While treating a chronic disease like RA, every effort is made to avoid creating a dependency upon narcotic analgesics. Some narcotics in small doses are acceptable and cannot be avoided, including propoxyphene (Darvon) or propoxyphene with acetaminophen (Darvocet N-100), codeine derivatives like hydrocodone (Vicodin), codeine with acetaminophen (Tylenol #3), tramadol (Ultram), or tramadol with acetaminophen (Ultracet). These medications are intended for people with moderate to moderately severe pain. Propoxyphene has weak analgesic properties and is occasionally associated with hallucinations in the elderly.

Anti-inflammatory Agents

Anti-inflammatory agents include aspirin (salicylates), nonsteroidal anti-inflammatory drugs (NSAIDs), or corticosteroids. Because of the added risk for side effects, these medications typically are not combined. Combining anti-inflammatories results in additive adverse events or the potential for double trouble. This is rarely worth the risk. Anti-inflammatories do not change the course of RA; they are symptomatic treatment only.

Anti-inflammatories provide relief of symptoms including redness, swelling, warmth, and pain. In low doses, all of the NSAIDs are pain relievers. They are prompt in onset, so that relief occurs within minutes or hours. Millions of Americans regularly use an NSAID. NSAIDs are popular because they are effective and relatively safe when taken properly. Like any other medication, they are not for everyone, cause side effects, and interact with other medications. The reduction of the signs of inflammation and pain takes several days. Most people believe there are no significant differences among all the available NSAIDs with regard to efficacy. There are some differences in the incidence of side effects and dose. Serum aspirin levels are measured to determine adequate dosing and compliance, but measurable NSAID levels are not available. To reduce upset stomach, NSAIDs are taken with food, rather than on an empty stomach. Patients demonstrating intolerance to this group of drugs require a concomitant gastrointestinal (GI) protective agent. Unfortunately, many patients with serious GI side effects from NSAIDs never develop noticeable symptoms. There is concern that the concomitant use of antacids or acid-blocking drugs will cover up the symptoms of an ulcer and increase the risk for GI bleeding secondary to NSAIDs.

The NSAIDs are divided into traditional NSAIDs and selective COX-2 inhibitors. Celecoxib (Celebrex), valdecoxib (Bextra), and rofecoxib (Vioxx) are the original COX-2 selective drugs approved for arthritis. COX-2 inhibitors are not more effective than traditional anti-inflammatories, but are safer for the GI tract. Rofecoxib (Vioxx), an early COX-2 selective drug, was withdrawn from the market because of concern for cardiovascular effects resulting in increased heart attacks and stroke as compared to traditional NSAIDs. Eventually, valdecoxib was also withdrawn. Valdecoxib was associated with an increased risk for a severe rash and cardiovascular problems in patients following heart surgery. Corticosteroids are the most potent anti-inflammatory medication, but they result in side effects not always acceptable. The side effects of corticosteroids are guaranteed to occur.

Remittive Drug Therapy

Long-acting antirheumatic drugs have the potential to slow the progression of the RA. They are not a cure. These medications are disease-modifying anti-rheumatic drugs (DMARDs), second-line agents, or slow-acting antirheumatic drugs. DMARDs include gold or chrysotherapy (Solganol, Aurolate), d-penicillamine (Depen, Cuprimine),

antimalarials like hydroxychloroquine (Plaquenil) or quinacrine (Atabrine), sulfasalazine (Azulfidine) and immunosuppressive, chemotherapeutic, or anti-cancer drugs like methotrexate (Rheumatrex, Trexall) or azathioprine (Imuran). Drugs suppressing rejection in organ transplantation are used and include cyclosporine (Neoral, Sandimmune). Newer medications include leflunomide (Arava) and biologicals like entanercept (Enbrel), adalimumab (Humira) and infliximab (Remicade). The immunoabsorption column (Prosorba column) was approved by the FDA for the treatment of moderate to severe adult RA in patients with longstanding disease who have failed or are intolerant of DMARDs. The column binds a silica matrix to a protein, which has the affinity to bind antibodies related to RA, but Prosorba column is cumbersome and expensive to use with limited effects. The standard course of treatment is twelve weekly outpatient sessions. Since the introduction of biologicals, many drug regimes have fallen out of favor. Injectable and oral gold is rarely used because of the superiority of other medications. D-penicillamine has also been found to be a less desirable DMARD.

There are a number of experimental medications currently in clinical investigation. New approaches to the therapy of RA are on the horizon. New therapies are important to patients who develop refractory RA, especially if the disease fails to respond adequately to prescribed treatments and runs a resistant course with progressive joint damage, deformity, and complications. The lack of a cure for RA and the inability to induce remissions with current drugs has led to the idea of combining DMARDs. These combinations are often effective therapy. Most drug treatment for RA works better with methotrexate than without, although the reason is not entirely understood. The goal of drug treatment in RA is to induce a complete remission, but how do you define a remission?

Interpreting Remission in Rheumatoid Arthritis

There are many ways to interpret improvement or remission of RA in response to medicine. An accurate definition is important in academic medicine during the comparison of different medications and their respective clinical efficacies. Physicians use a multitude of clinical and laboratory signs and symptoms during therapeutic decision-making in the management of RA. There is probably no right or wrong answer. DMARD medications only maintain remissions. Permanent remissions are unusual. Even so, complete remission remains the goal of RA treatment. There is an occasional patient who goes into a spontaneous remission, regardless of interventions. Burned-out RA occurs occasionally in older individuals experiencing a remission after longstanding disease. Rheumatic illnesses are characterized

by good and bad times. These cycles are not necessarily true and permanent remissions. These periods of time last days, weeks, or months. At the onset of disease, an individual needs to be given a period of weeks to determine whether a spontaneous remission will occur without the need for drug therapy. At least some or all of the following criteria are necessary to define a remission.

Remission Criteria for Rheumatoid Arthritis

- ◊ no progression of bone changes (erosions) or joint space narrowing on an x-ray
- ◊ a response by the patient that reports improved quality of life and better function, especially with activities of daily living or work
- ◊ the need for fewer concomitant medications, especially steroids, narcotics, and other drug therapy with side effects
- ◊ improvement of laboratory studies and inflammatory markers
- ◊ physician evidence of no swollen or tender joints

Measurements of Improvement in Rheumatoid Arthritis

Other findings in RA include constitutional symptoms like fatigue or weight loss. An assessment of functional status, a measure of overall assessment by the physician or by the patient, is an important criterion to measure activity of disease and the response to treatment. Extra-articular manifestations of RA significantly affect prognosis and the severity of disease and ultimately the institution and extent of treatment. Their improvement suggests control of the inflammation of the disease.

Some patients will do well with one form of remittive therapy and not another. It is unfortunate, but there is no way to predict who will do well or who will have problems. There is no simple test that will predict a response or a side effect to the drugs. Remittive therapy needs to be initiated and monitored carefully.

Disease Activity Score (DAS)

DAS is a measurement often used in clinical practice to measure the benefits of RA therapy. It is accurate, practical, and relatively simple. The DAS 44 measures forty-four different joints while the modified DAS, or DAS 28, counts the twenty-eight tender and swollen joints of the shoulders, elbows, wrists, hands, and knees. The number is then put into a formula that also takes advantage of the erythrocyte sedimentation rate and an objective measurement by the patient. The ease of use of the DAS makes it possible to collect valuable informa-

tion about disease activity of a patient in daily clinical practice. Treatment decisions are based on an objective assessment and the change in disease activity. The Disease Activity Score (DAS) was developed to evaluate the clinical picture of rheumatoid arthritis at a particular point in time.

Disease Activity Score

	DAS44	DAS28
High Disease Score	>3.7	>5.1
Low Disease Score	<2.4	<3.2
Clinical Remission	<1.6	<2.6

ACR Response Criteria

Currently the best evaluation tool is the American College of Rheumatology Response Criteria (ACR Response). This is recognized by the FDA as the best clinical measurement of rheumatoid disease in clinical drug trials. An ACR response is defined as 20 percent, 50 percent, or 70 percent response in the following parameters:

◊ improvement in swollen joint count,

◊ improvement in tender joint count, and

... and improvement in at least three of the following five measures:

◊ patient's global assessment
◊ physician's global assessment
◊ patient's assessment of pain
◊ acute-phase reactant
◊ disability (HAQ)

The ACR response criteria do not necessarily reflect all clinically useful information. Since it is an expression of change over time, the ACR response criteria cannot be used to evaluate a patient's disease activity at any given moment.

Principles of Remission in Rheumatoid Arthritis

Regardless of the best definition of remission, there are several important principles to understand. A reduction in the erythrocyte sedimentation rate (ESR) after treatment indicates less inflammation and a response to treatment. This is a simple and relatively inexpensive test utilized in medicine for more than seventy years. Laboratories tend to use several different methods for this test. Most experts prefer the Westergren method. The ESR remains convenient, continues to be inexpensive, and enjoys familiarity with most physicians. However, it remains nonspecific and is elevated in other inflammatory states like infection, malignancy, or other rheumatic illnesses. The C-reactive protein (CRP) is another indicator of inflammation measured in the blood and is more sensitive than the ESR.

Since the CRP indicates an interruption in the inflammatory process, the CRP has some importance in monitoring the actual disease process. These two laboratory tests are nonspecific indicators of inflammation and fail to help differentiate RA from other forms of arthritis or other rheumatic illnesses. The importance of these tests is to monitor the clinical disease activity in patients with RA. Persistent elevations of these tests correlate positively with joint destruction. Improvement of inflammatory indicators is objective evidence of a beneficial response to treatment. The rheumatoid factor is not significantly affected by treatment and doesn't have a value in monitoring response.

A reduced need for anti-inflammatories suggests a response to treatment. Decreasing daily corticosteroids just a few milligrams is important and diminishes side effects. The need for fewer NSAIDs and pain medications is important. Effective treatment with NSAIDs is usually not associated with a significant change in the ESR or CRP.

The patient's subjective interpretation of improvement includes the duration of pain and morning stiffness. Morning stiffness is a nonspecific complaint of reduced mobility of the joints upon arising in the morning. Morning stiffness is measured in minutes or hours, or it can last all day. Stiffness suggests worse disease activity and indicates synovitis or inflammation around the joints. Practically, synovitis is determined by a good physical exam by the physician, but future clinical tests, including ultrasound or MR, will be more sensitive. In most cases, a complete remission is not achieved. The management of RA is to control the progression of disease activity, alleviate pain, maintain activities of daily living, maximize quality of life, and slow the rate of joint damage.

Principles of Rheumatoid Arthritis Management
◊ control progression of systemic disease
◊ alleviate pain
◊ maintain activities of daily living
◊ maximize quality of life
◊ slow radiographic progression

CHAPTER THREE

Osteoporosis

Fractures of the spine and hip are major obstacles to a normal quality of life. The related suffering, expense, and inconvenience for patients and family members cannot be measured in a meaningful way. Studies have shown that 15 to 25 percent of elderly women who sustain a fractured hip will lose their independence within the first year after the fracture. The estimated cost of hip fractures in the United States is at least six to eight billion dollars a year. If the incidence of such fractures could be decreased, the cost savings to society would be substantial. Osteoporosis is a common disease. It is estimated that more than 50 percent of postmenopausal women will be affected. In women, the incidence of osteoporosis is greater than heart attack, breast cancer, and stroke combined. More than one million individuals in America suffer osteoporotic fractures each year. During a woman's lifetime, she will lose an average of 30 to 50 percent of her body's bone density. Four in ten women older than fifty years of age are likely to suffer an osteoporosis-related fracture of the hip, spine, or wrist at some point during the remainder of their lifetimes. Men are not protected from osteoporosis or fractures. Low testosterone levels lead to osteoporosis. The treatment of prostate cancer can increase the risk for fracture. The use of any corticosteroid treatment for any medical condition decreases bone strength.

Osteoporosis simply means having too little density in the bones. This leads to weak, fragile bones, and fractures. The bone becomes more porous. After the mid-thirties, bone loss becomes continuous as a part of the aging process. The greatest bone density achieved is the peak bone mass. This occurs at different ages, but is usually achieved by age thirty. The level of bone density at which bone fractures occur much more readily is the fracture threshold. This occurs from bone loss or developing less peak bone mass initially.

Minor falls or fragility falls from standing height can cause fractures of the wrist, hip, spine, or pelvis in men or women with osteoporosis. Repeated spinal fractures result in compression fractures of vertebral bodies and reduced height. In the U.S., more than seven hundred thousand vertebral compression fractures are diagnosed yearly. Most spinal fractures do not cause symptoms, yet 20 percent of these people will have a second vertebral fracture within one year of the first spinal fracture. Repeated spinal fractures result in a kyphotic deformity of the upper thoracic spine (dowager's or widow's hump). Vertebral fractures result in loss of height of several inches, difficulty with clothes fitting normally, and chronic pain. Height loss may indicate an unsuspected spinal fracture in an individual and be an important signal for osteoporosis. Women and men who break a bone due to osteoporosis are more likely to have another fracture—of the spine, hip, or shoulder—during the next five years. Most subsequent fractures occur in the first year after the initial broken bone.

Risk Factors of Osteoporosis

A family history of osteoporosis increases one's risk of osteoporosis. There is a greater risk with low body weight, smoking, low dietary calcium intake, excess alcohol, and high caffeine consumption. If you are a non-black woman, your chance of developing osteoporosis during your lifetime is about 25 percent. If estrogen replacement therapy is begun as soon as the menstrual cycle stops, this risk can be cut in half. Bone loss is most rapid during the first few years after menopause and then declines slowly with age. A variety of medical treatments promotes bone loss, including systemic steroids, thyroid, or anticonvulsant therapy. Early menopause occurring naturally, prematurely, or as a result of oophorectomy results in bone loss. Immediate estrogen replacement therapy benefits bone. Many women are now avoiding estrogen. The only clear-cut indication for estrogen replacement after menopause is not osteoporosis, but uncontrolled vasomotor symptoms like hot flashes. Celiac disease is characterized by chronic bowel inflammation and affects approximately one million Americans. Classic symptoms include diarrhea and abdominal cramps. Calcium and vitamin D are both malabsorbed. Many patients with celiac disease do not have bowel symptoms and only present after a fracture related to osteoporosis. The BMD is decreased. Sensitive blood tests detect celiac disease and allow early treatment. Most patients respond to a gluten-free diet. Other medical conditions like kidney disease, endocrine disease, and excess thyroid hormone replacement are associated with osteoporosis. Men with low levels of testosterone (hypogonadism) develop osteoporosis. Other less common illnesses are also associated with osteoporosis.

Measuring Bone Density

There is an indirect relationship between the density of bones and risk for fracture. A bone mineral density (BMD) test determines risk for fracture. Dual energy x-ray absorbtiometry (DXA) is a fast, simple, convenient means to determine the bone density measurement. It is painless and is done without the need for the patient to undress. Insurance companies, health maintenance organizations (HMOs), and Medicare recognize and reimburse for bone density measurements.

Bone density measurements detect low bone density before a fracture occurs, predict the chance of a fracture in the future, confirm the diagnosis of osteoporosis, determine the rate of bone loss, and monitor the effects of treatment at periodic intervals.

A standard x-ray provides a crude measurement of BMD. At least 30 percent of bone mass must be gone before it is detected by x-ray. A BMD by DXA is much more precise, accurate, and requires only about one-thirtieth the radiation of a standard chest x-ray. A central BMD test measures BMD at the spine

---

Who Needs Bone Density Testing

◊ all women aged sixty-five and older
◊ all men aged seventy and older
◊ anyone with a fragility fracture
◊ anyone with a disease, condition, or medication associated with osteoporosis, especially steroids
◊ anyone considering therapy for osteoporosis, if bone density testing would facilitate the decision
◊ women who have been on hormone replacement therapy for prolonged periods
◊ anyone treated for osteoporosis to monitor therapy

Medicare Reimbursement for BMD Testing

◊ estrogen deficient women undecided about hormones
◊ individuals with spinal or x-ray evidence of bone loss
◊ anyone taking long-term steroid treatment
◊ primary hyperparathyroidism with no symptoms
◊ monitoring of therapy for osteoporosis.

or hip. This is done by DXA technology. DXA uses a small dose of x-ray to measure BMD. DXA is the gold standard for measurement of bone density and is preferred both for diagnosing osteoporosis and monitoring the effects of therapy. Central testing of the spine is done by quantitative computerized tomography (QCT). This scanning utilizes large doses of x-ray and is less available than in the past, because of the superiority of DXA scanning.

Peripheral BMD tests measure other skeletal sites, such as the heel or forearm, and use a variety of technologies including peripheral DXA (pDXA), quantitative ultrasound (QUS), and peripheral QCT scanning (pQCT). Peripheral tests are used to estimate the risk of fracture, but they are not recommended to diagnose osteoporosis or to monitor the effects of therapy. It is recommended that a central bone density test be done. The BMD acts as a surrogate marker to identify individuals at risk for osteoporosis as well as a to measure response to therapy.

Criteria for Osteoporosis

The World Health Organization (WHO) defines osteoporosis as a T-score equal to or less than -2.5 deviations below a young adult female when done on a DXA scan. The T-score is a method for comparing the bone density of an individual to that of a healthy person at age thirty. A T-score of zero is normal.

The lower or more negative the T-score, the greater the risk for fracture. The criteria are established for postmenopausal women, so it is difficult to compare T-scores to other groups, like men or children.

A fragility fracture is a broken bone resulting from no, or minimal, trauma, such as falling to the floor from the standing position. Fragility fractures define osteoporosis. It is better to discover osteoporosis by measuring BMD before a fracture occurs. A low BMD by DXA, multiple risk factors for osteoporosis, or a fracture provides an opportunity for immediate treatment to lower the risk of future fracture. After an osteoporotic fracture, treatment lowers the risk of having a subsequent fracture. Once a fragility fracture occurs, it is pertinent that a DXA scan is done to determine the need for treatment.

Definition of Osteoporosis
◊ T-score <-2.5
◊ fragility fracture

Turnover of Bone

Quality of bone is a more important issue than quantity of bone as measured by DXA. Bone is dynamic and constantly being laid down (formation) and broken down (reabsorption). Accelerated bone turnover of this coupled process is an important reason to develop osteoporosis and fracture. Laboratory studies have been developed to measure the breakdown products, including both serum and urinary measurements. Elevated levels of these markers indicate high bone turnover or absorption. Similarly, there are a number of markers, such as bone alkaline phosphate and osteocalcin, that reflect an individual's formation potential. Measurements of both markers can help identify at-risk patients, appropriate therapy, compliance, and response to therapy.

Hormonal Replacement Therapy (HRT)

Women with trace or undetectable estrogen levels in the blood are at a 2.5 times greater relative risk for osteoporosis and debilitating bone and hip fractures than other post-menopausal women. Therefore, estrogen replacement therapy (ERT) at the time of menopause can positively impact bone loss and is one of the most effective means of preventing fracture from osteoporosis. The findings in a large national study, the Women's Health Initiative (WHI), questioned the safety of estrogens. The study enrolled sixteen thousand healthy postmenopausal women and reported increased risk of heart attack, stroke, invasive breast cancer, pulmonary emboli, and thrombosis of the legs in postmenopausal women fifty to seventy-nine years of age. During the

five years of treatment with oral estrogens (Premarin) 0.625 milligrams combined with progesterone (Provera) 2.5 milligrams relative to placebo, estrogen reduced the risk of hip fractures by 34 percent. The increased risks for adverse effects resulted in many women discontinuing estrogen, unless they experience moderate to severe hot flashes or flushing during menopause. In these same women, estrogen had been delaying the usual bone loss effects of menopause. After years of ERT, once estrogen is discontinued, bone loss occurs at a rapid rate, as if menopause occurred without estrogen replacement. Women with undetectable estrogen blood levels are at a significant risk for osteoporosis and hip fractures.

Estradiol Transdermal Patches

Estradiol transdermal patches (Menostar) at fourteen micrograms per day delivers a low dose of plant-derived estrogen that can be used in women with or without a uterus. Menostar is a clear, dime-sized, once-a-week patch that delivers half the dose per day of the lowest currently available dose of transdermal estrogen therapy for postmenopausal osteoporosis prevention. This patch does not require a daily or monthly concomitant progestin to protect against endometrial cancer among women with an intact uterus. In clinical studies, there was no difference in the number of incidents of breast cancer, blood clots, or cardiovascular events in the study group as compared to placebo. Low-dose estradiol transdermal patches improve bone mass, but there have been no studies to prove that the fracture rate diminishes in those individual at risk. Estrogen therapy should not be used in individuals with any of the following conditions.

Reasons Not to Use Estrogen

- ◊ abnormal uterine bleeding
- ◊ history of uterine cancer
- ◊ history of breast cancer
- ◊ estrogen-dependent cancer
- ◊ blood clots
- ◊ stroke or heart attacks
- ◊ pregnancy
- ◊ liver disease
- ◊ concern for any of the above

Diet and Supplements

Calcium

Calcium in the amount of one thousand to fifteen hundred milligrams daily, or about six ounces of yogurt, one cup of calcium-fortified orange juice, and two ounces of hard cheese to supplement diets low in calcium, is recommended. The best natural sources of calcium are dairy products, including whole or skim milk and cheese. Leafy green vegetables, including broccoli, collards, turnip greens, mustard greens, and spinach are also good sources. Salmon, sardines, and raw oysters are high in calcium too. The recommended daily allowance (RDA) of calcium for women age nineteen and older is one thousand milligrams, but many experts feel this is not enough for women after menopause and recommend as much as fifteen hundred milligrams daily after menopause to reduce the risk of osteoporosis. Most women get about five hundred to six hundred milligrams of calcium in their daily diet, so without supplements, there is an increased risk for osteoporosis. For these reasons, many women should consider adding calcium tablets to their daily routine. Very high consumption of calcium increases the risk for kidney stones, especially in those individuals with a prior history of kidney stones. Less than two thousand milligrams daily of calcium constitutes a very small risk for kidney stones.

Calcium carbonate has a higher percentage of elemental calcium in each tablet than other supplements. It is the easiest calcium to find in the stores and the most affordable. Calcium carbonate causes gas or constipation. Since stomach acid is required to absorb it, calcium carbonate is taken with or immediately after a meal. Calcium citrate already contains acid, so it doesn't require stomach acid for absorption. It doesn't need to be taken with food and it does not cause constipation.

Vitamin D

Vitamin D promotes the process of bone formation. While calcium and other minerals are the building blocks of healthy bones, it is vitamin D that regulates calcium's actions in the body and makes calcium available for absorption into bone. Vitamin D is produced in the skin with the help of sunlight and is easily obtained from the diet as well. This vitamin is made in response to sun exposure. Indoor jobs, sedentary lifestyles, fear of skin cancer, and long winter months leave many women deficient of vitamin D. However, several minutes of sun exposure a few times a week in the winter months adds significant equivalents of vitamin D to the body. Milk, margarine, and many other foods are fortified with vitamin D. It occurs naturally in significant amounts in eggs, liver, and fish. Adequate amounts of vitamin D should be consumed daily. Vitamin D needs to be present in the diet on a regular basis along with calcium to perform its functions. The RDA of vitamin D is four hundred international units (IU). Concentrated forms and supplements of vitamin D can result in vitamin D toxicity, yet on occasion, eight hundred IUs are recommended. Almost all multivitamin tablets contain four hundred IUs of vitamin D.

Bisphosphonates

Like other organ systems, once bone is formed, it is still very much alive. Besides its supportive nature, bone acts as a reserve or bank for calcium. Each day, osteoblast cells make bone (formation) and osteoclast cells take bone away (reabsorption) to regulate calcium. Bisphosphonate drugs block reabsorption of bone by interfering with osteoclasts. Osteoblasts build bone and strengthen it. The process of bone formation and bone reabsorption is coupled with the activity of the osteoblasts and osteoclasts respectively. Interfering with one portion of the process interferes with the other. The benefits are monitored by using the DXA scan and measuring the BMD. Oral bisphosphonates are poorly absorbed and must be taken first thing in the morning on an empty stomach, with no food taken thereafter for a minimum of one-half hour. Food or other pills decrease absorption in the stomach. Bisphosphonates have been associated with esophagitis. It is recommended that all bisphosphonates be taken after awakening in the morning while in an upright position and out of bed. They should be accompanied by a full glass of water to minimize esophageal irritation. In this way, they are well tolerated. An occasional patient experiences bone pain, aggravation of arthritic complaints, and abdominal pain that will usually resolve themselves. Individuals with moderate to severe kidney disease should not take bisphosphonates.

Bisphosphonates are approved for the prevention and treatment of postmenopausal osteoporosis in women and all patients receiving chronic cortico-steroids. Oral alendronate (Fosamax), risidronate (Actonel), and ibandronate (Boniva) are FDA approved bisphosphonates for the treatment of osteoporosis. Ibandronate is more potent than the other bisphosphonates and shows extended effects for a month. Oral etidronate (Didronel) is indicated for Paget's disease, but it has been used for osteoporosis in a complicated dose schedule. Intravenous pamidronate (Aredia) and zoledronate (Zometa) are indicated to treat elevated levels of calcium or bone metastasis secondary to cancer or bone, but are useful for their prolonged beneficial effect on osteoporosis. Intravenous ibandronate has been approved to be given every three months.

Oral risidronate at 2.5 or 5 milligrams daily reduces the incidence of new vertebral fractures almost 50 percent in postmenopausal women already at severe risk for another spinal fracture because of existing spinal fractures. To improve compliance, weekly 35-milligram dosing was studied and found to result in similar BMD improvements at the lumbar spine and hip. There is a perception that residronate may have less gastrointestinal adverse effects than similar other medications. Oral alendronate at 5 or 10 milligrams daily also has the ability to reduce bone loss and decrease the incidence of fracture about 50 percent in people with low bone density measurements, regardless of preceding fractures. The knowledge of the prolonged effects of alendronate and compliance issues of daily dosing lead to the utilization of 70 milligrams once a week. Studies subsequently proved equal efficacy on BMD compared to daily dosing. Data now suggests that risidronate and alendronate can be discontinued for twelve to twenty-four months after a period of time as a drug holiday with maintenance of BMD benefit. The effect this has on fracture reduction is unclear. Monthly dosing of ibandronate appears to be just as effective as daily dosing of bisphosphonates. Monthly dosing potentially improves compliance. Adverse events with ibandronate are similar to other bisphosphonates.

Calcitonin

Calcitonin is given as a subcutaneous injection (Calcimar) or nasal spray (Miacalcin). This naturally occurring hormone blocks resorption of bone and has been useful in relieving the pain of acute vertebral compression fractures. The spray is used more often than the subcutaneous injection. One spray is directed into one nostril once a day. In controlled studies, calcitonin decreased the risk of vertebral fractures by about 54 percent, but studies to demonstrate the effects on other bone fractures have not been done. Calcitonin is prescribed for women who are at least five years postmenopausal and are unable to tolerate or refuse other osteoporosis medications. The nasal spray can cause nasal irritation and headaches.

Selective Estrogen Replacement Modulators (SERMs)

Raloxifene (Evista) is not an estrogen. Raloxifene is a selective estrogen receptor modulator (SERM). SERMs help build bone without negatively affecting the breast or uterus. The FDA has approved raloxifene for use in the prevention of postmenopausal osteoporosis. These nontraditional hormones are sometimes referred to as designer estrogens. Raloxifene acts like estrogen in certain tissues, but not in others. Raloxifene increases BMD as measured by DXA, though not as well as estrogen does. The effects on decreasing fractures have been beneficial and proven at the spine. Because raloxifene acts selectively, most women do not experience the vaginal bleeding, bloating, and breast tenderness associated with estrogen. Raloxifene does not help the symptoms of hot flashes, insomnia, or mood swings. SERMs may precipitate hot flashes or flushing.

There is no evidence for preventing hip fracture with SERMs, although it may still have that beneficial effect. In clinical trials, raloxifene lowers total cholesterol by about 7 percent and LDL (bad cholesterol) about 11 percent. It does not change HDL (good cholesterol). Raloxifene does not increase the risk of breast or uterine cancer. It has not been established if raloxifene is able to reduce the risk of breast cancer, although that is a keen area of research. Most of the side effects are mild and usually do not cause women to stop taking the medication. The most common side effects of raloxifene are hot flashes and leg cramps. Hot flashes are more common during the first six months of treatment. Women who already have hot flashes can still take raloxifene; however, raloxifene may aggravate their hot flashes. Raloxifene is taken only after menopause and is not to be taken if there is a history of blood clotting, congestive heart failure, cancer, or liver disease.

While taking raloxifene, periods of immobility must be avoided. Immobility like prolonged travel increases the risk of blood clots. Raloxifene adds to the risk. Raloxifene should be discontinued at least three days before a planned surgery or prolonged immobility. Taking 81 milligrams of aspirin once daily decreases the chance for blood clots. Raloxifene is then restarted when normal activities resume. Any form of estrogen therapy that comes as a pill, patch, or injection should not be taken at the same time as raloxifene. Tests to monitor anticoagulation therapy may be effected while taking raloxifene.

Parathyroid Hormone (PTH)

Hyperparathyroidism results in continuous elevated levels of parathyroid hormone (PTH) and causes bone loss and osteoporosis. The intermittent use of PTH has the opposite effect on the bone as the continuous effect of elevated PTH levels. The use of intermittent recombinant human parathyroid hormone (teriparatide) represents a significant treatment for osteoporosis. Teriparatide (Forteo) increases bone density in contrast to the effects of hyperparathyroidism. Except for teriparatide, all other FDA-approved therapies act by inhibiting bone resorption during its remodeling process and the bone turnover of the skeleton. No previous therapy directly increases bone density. Teriparatide is a powerful bone builder that accelerates the turnover of bone. Its effect is greater on bone formation than resorption. The net result is greater BMD, as well as reduction of fracture risk at both vertebral and nonvertebral sites. Teriparatide increases the BMD more than all other therapies. Vertebral risk fracture is reduced in more than half the patients, and as many are less likely to have a new nonvertebral fragility fracture. Teriparatide is indicated for postmenopausal women and men who are a high risk for fracture, including those people with a history of a prior osteoporotic fracture, a history of multiple risk factors for future fracture, or those individuals who have failed or are intolerant of other osteoporosis therapies.

Teriparatide represents the available form of parathyroid hormone and is a daily self-injectable therapy. The decision to change therapy or use teriparatide should be based upon good sound medical advice. Stable BMD reduces the risk for fracture. If the loss of BMD on current therapy is outside the potential error of the DXA equipment, a change in therapy may be appropriate. Other causes of bone loss should be explored: vitamin D deficiency, celiac disease, hyperparathyroidism, myeloma and others. It is unclear if there are added benefits to combining teriparatide with therapies like alendronate, risidronate, and ibandronate or in sequence.

Teriparatide is given as daily self-injections using a small unique pen device that contains a month of therapy. The needle is discarded daily and a new one attached. Injection sites are prepped with an alcohol wipe prior to the insertion of the needle. The injection sites are rotated around the abdomen or upper leg. A small sting is associated with the injection.

The adverse effects of teriparatide are relatively infrequent and not serious. Teriparatide is generally safe. Studies in rats at doses much greater than ever utilized in humans revealed the development of cancer (osteosarcoma). This has never been reported in humans as a result of teriparatide use. The skeleton of the rats is distinctly different from that of humans, and this explains the risk for the development of cancer. Even so, the FDA has insisted that this medicine not be prescribed in those individuals at risk for osteosarcoma, including those with Paget's bone disease, a history of prior radiation therapy, bone cancer, metastasis of cancer to bone, elevated blood calcium, and hyperparathyroidism. The duration of teriparatide therapy is limited to twenty-four months.

Indications for Teriparatide
◊   men or postmenopausal women at significant risk for fracture
◊   prior osteoporotic fracture, especially multiple spinal fractures
◊   severe osteoporosis (low T-score and fracture)
◊   multiple risk factors for future fracture
◊   individuals intolerant or who have failed other therapies

Other Treatments for Osteoporosis

Thiazide diuretics minimize the loss of calcium in the urine and are helpful in some people. Other treatments under investigation include powerful forms of vitamin D, newer forms of sodium fluoride, strontium ranelate, and anti-estrogen drugs. Oral strontium stimulates bone formation and reduces the resorption of bone, but it has not yet been approved for the treatment of osteoporosis. Further synthetic parathyroid hormone treatments are expected in the future.

Spinal Fractures

Traditionally, vertebral compression fractures have been treated with bed rest, medication, and back bracing. This approach relieves the pain, but leaves the spine in its deformed state. Balloon kyphoplasty is a surgical management of vertebral body compression fractures. Kyphoplasty is minimally invasive and relieves the back pain of acute spinal fractures. Kyphoplasty addresses both the deformity and pain by stabilizing the fracture and correcting the vertebral deformity. The kyphoplasty procedure is done in the hospital or as an outpatient procedure under general or local anesthesia. Under the guidance of x-ray, a small percutaneous tube is placed into the area of the fracture. The tube provides a path for the insertion of a balloon. When inflated, the balloon raises the collapsed fractured bone and creates a space inside the vertebral body. The balloon is then removed and the space filled with cement to support the bone. Filling the space prevents further collapse of the vertebral fracture and provides pain relief within hours. The procedure typically takes less than one hour per fracture. Once completed, the patient needs to return to a physician for further medical management of osteoporosis. If left untreated, spinal deformities lead to subsequent fractures and loss of height and kyphosis. The compression of the chest and abdominal cavity because of severe kyphosis leads to chronic debilitating pain, decreasing lung function, impaired physical function, a protuberant abdomen, early satiety, decreased activities of daily living, chronic anxiety, and depression.

A similar procedure is vertebroplasty. Vertebroplasty is done by the radiologist with local anesthesia. A catheter is inserted into the area of fracture through the skin percutaneously without a balloon. Cement is then injected directly into the area of the fracture. An unfortunate aspect of this procedure is that vertebroplasty doesn't allow as much control of the cement and where it is going as kyphoplasty does. The vertebroplasty doesn't re-inflate the compressed vertebral body, but it can provide immediate pain relief.

The key to the management of spinal fractures is not treatment after a fracture occurs, but prevention. Regular exercise reduces the risk of fractures by preventing both osteoporosis and falls. Exercise improves gait, balance, coordination, and muscle strength. Exercise should be part of the strategy for all individuals with osteoporosis. Good lifestyle habits like avoiding smoking and eating will make a difference.

Steroid-Induced Osteoporosis

The association between the use of corticosteroids and bone loss is well established. An estimated 30 to 50 percent of patients on chronic corticosteroid therapy experience an osteoporotic fracture. The treatment of many forms of arthritis and other illnesses require chronic corticosteroids. These same patients are at significant risk for osteoporosis and fracture. The continuous use of corticosteroids requires measures to prevent osteoporosis, its effects on the bones, and the risk for fracture. It is important to assess one's risk for fracture if corticosteroids are going to be utilized for any illness. Even a short duration of corticosteroid therapy has a deleterious effect on the BMD. The risk of vertebral fracture is five times greater in patients receiving 7.5 milligrams of prednisone daily compared to patients not taking prednisone. All individuals committed to oral corticosteroid therapy for more than three months, regardless of dose, should be assessed for the risk of osteoporosis and fracture by measuring BMD. The early months of corticosteroid therapy are associated with increased bone loss. All patients should have primary prevention immediately. As much as 10 to 20 percent of bone mass is lost in the first few months of therapy with corticosteroids. Besides being assessed for low BMD, individuals at increased risk for fracture are identified by reviewing other risk factors, including previous fragility fractures or vertebral fractures. All individuals, regardless of age, initiating oral corticosteroids with an equivalent dose of prednisone 5 milligrams daily or more for at least three months need a bisphosphonate drug as preventive therapy. A baseline BMD is done and the patient supplemented with calcium and vitamin D. Future corticosteroid doses and duration of therapy in these same individuals

Burden of Osteoporosis
◊ Calcium is critically important for healthy bones.
◊ Vitamin D is required for bone formation.
◊ Daily physical activity is crucial to building strong bone.
◊ Annually 1.2 million people have osteoporotic fractures.
◊ Risk of fracture increases with age for women.
◊ Osteoporosis takes a significant toll on society.
◊ Diet and physical activity make the difference between a frail and a strong skeleton.
◊ Osteoporosis can be avoided.
◊ At-risk individuals must be identified and treated.
◊ BMD is the "gold standard" for identifying those at risk.
◊ Bone strength is related to BMD.
◊ Drug therapy should be considered in all individuals who have osteoporosis.

is minimized to lessen bone loss. Lowering corticosteroid doses periodically, stopping therapy, or adding alternative drug therapy that helps lower corticosteroid doses benefits the bones. However, the corticosteroid dose must still be adequate to treat the underlying illness.

Bone Breakers

Alcohol disrupts calcium balance and interferes with the action of vitamin D. The risk of hip fracture is 55 percent higher in smokers. Excess thyroid hormone aggravates osteoporosis. Lithium and some anticonvulsants interfere with vitamin D. Prolonged bed rest, inactivity, and lack of exercise all contribute to decreased bone density.

CHAPTER FOUR

Systemic Lupus Erythematosis (Lupus)

Lupus is a chronic autoimmune disease, which results in inflammation of multiple areas of the body, especially the skin, joints, blood, and kidney. It is the inflammation of tissues that results in the symptoms of lupus. The illness affects young women of the childbearing years, between fifteen to forty-five years of age. It is estimated that 1.5 million Americans have lupus. The elderly or young are not excluded. Nine women get lupus for every one man that gets the disease. Although lupus occurs within families, there is no known gene, or genes, which are thought to cause the illness. A small percentage of patients will have a close relative that already has or may develop lupus. An even smaller percentage of the children born to individuals with lupus will develop the illness. Ten percent of people with lupus have a close relative that has, or will develop, lupus. Only about 5 percent of children born to people with lupus will develop the illness. Lupus is often called a woman's disease, despite the fact that many men are affected. The symptoms of the disease are the same in men and women. People of African, American Indian, and Asian origin are thought to develop the disease more frequently than Caucasian women.

Hormonal factors may explain why lupus occurs more frequently in females than in males. The increase of disease symptoms before menstrual periods and/or during pregnancy support the belief that hormones, particularly estrogen, may be involved. The exact hormonal reason for the greater prevalence of lupus in women and the cyclic increase in symptoms is unknown. There is no reason for lupus patients to avoid birth control pills during their fertile years or estrogen replacement therapy during menopause.

The Immune Response

The immune system normally makes proteins (antibodies) to protect the body against viruses, bacteria, and other foreign materials (antigens). In an autoimmune disorder such as lupus, the immune system loses its ability to tell the difference between foreign substances (antigens) and its own cells and tissues (self). The immune system then makes antibodies directed against self. These auto-antibodies react with the self-antigens to form immune complexes. In lupus, these immune complexes deposit in the tissues and create inflammation, injury, and pain. Over 70 percent of patients with lupus have systemic disease. In systemic disease, antibodies deposit in different areas of the body. Of people with lupus, about one-half deposit antibodies that damage internal organs and one-half deposit antibodies outside the internal organs.

More people have lupus than have better-recognized diseases like AIDS, cerebral palsy, multiple sclerosis, sickle-cell anemia, and cystic fibrosis combined. A number of other diseases are closely related or may be part of lupus, including mixed connective tissue disease (MCTD), scleroderma or progressive systemic sclerosis (PSS), polymyositis (PM), dermatomyositis (DM), rheumatoid arthritis (RA), and Sjogren's syndrome (SS). About 5 percent of lupus patients have an overlap syndrome or a combination of symptoms of these related illnesses.

Clinical Course of Lupus

For the most part, lupus is a mild disease affecting only a few organs, but it may cause serious and life-threatening problems. It is helpful to think of the disease as a long railroad track or ladder, with the more serious manifestations of the disease like nephritis or cerebritis at one end of the track or ladder and minor symptoms like rash or joint pain at the other end. Joint pain without swelling (arthralgia) is a prominent part of the disease. There are a number of people who seem to have one foot on the railroad track and the other on shaky ground. These individuals are difficult to diagnose. Some have an ill-defined connective disease that may blossom to lupus at sometime or another. Close monitoring of these individuals is important. The disease is characterized by remissions (inactivity) and exacerbations (flares). Individuals can move up and down the railroad track in either direction over weeks, months, or years.

Although lupus affects any organ system of the body, most people experience symptoms in only a few organs. Many of the symptoms mimic other illnesses and are sometimes vague. The disease is characterized by a fluctuating and unpredictable course, and this makes lupus difficult to recognize. The diagnosis is made by a careful review of an individual's medical history, an analysis of the results obtained in routine laboratory tests, and specialized tests related to the patient's immune status. Currently, there is no single laboratory test that can determine whether a person has lupus. The antinuclear antibody (ANA) is a serological marker for autoimmunity. It is widely accepted as a screening test for lupus. Some researchers suggest lupus is on the increase; however, there is more likely a greater awareness. In combination with the awareness of lupus, symptoms, and the utilization of the ANA, the diagnosis is established earlier. The ANA is detectable in virtually all people with lupus and is the best initial diagnostic test to identify lupus. If the test is negative, the patient most likely does not have lupus.

Criteria to Establish Lupus

The American College of Rheumatology (ACR) has provided a list of eleven symptoms or signs that help distinguish lupus from other diseases. A person should have four or more of these criteria to be labeled with the diagnosis of lupus. The symptoms do not all have to occur at the same time. A person has SLE if any four or more of the eleven criteria are present. A detectable ANA by itself is not diagnostic of lupus, since the test is also detectable in other conditions.

The ANA test is reported as positive or negative. If positive, the results include a titer. The titer indicates how many times an individual's blood must be diluted to get a sample free of antinuclear antibodies. Typically, the laboratory technician begins with diluting the blood 1:20, then 1:40, 1:80, 1:160, 1:320, 1:640, 1:1280 and so on. A titer of 1:640 has greater concentration of antinuclear antibodies than a titer of 1:320 or 1:160. The test does not determine activity of disease and should be utilized as a marker of disease and not as a determinant of the need for therapy. The higher titers do have importance. Patients with active lupus have an ANA that is high in titer.

Laboratory tests that measure complement levels in the blood are also of some value. Complement is a circulating blood protein that combines with antibodies to destroy antigens. Complement is an amplifier of the immune system. If the total complement level is low, it suggests that antigen-antibody complexes have combined with complement and are being deposited in the tissues. If complement is being consumed in these immune complexes, the disease process is usually active and requires treatment. Other markers of disease include the autoantibodies anti-DNA, anti-Sm, anti-RNP, and anti-Ro. The anti-DNA correlates to activity of disease in SLE and is helpful in determining the need for treatment. Skin biopsies of both a lupus rash and normal skin help diagnose lupus. The interpretation of these tests is frequently difficult.

Anemia is the most common abnormality of lupus. About one-half of the patients are anemic. There are several reasons for anemia, including impaired kidney function, bleeding, inflammation at the site of red blood cell production in the bone marrow, and the premature destruction of red blood cells as a result of antibodies directed against red cells in the circulation. In patients with kidney failure, an injectable red cell stimulating hormone erythropoietin (Procrit, Epogen) helps stimulate production of red blood cells.

Low platelet counts (thrombocytopenia) results in excessive bruising and bleeding. Bleeding tendencies are aggravated by the use of aspirin, since aspirin inhibits platelet aggregation. The aspirin effect on platelets lasts the lifetime of platelets, usually several days after aspirin is stopped. NSAIDs have the same effect on the platelets, but only while NSAIDs are being taken. The COX-2 anti-inflammatories do not have an effect on platelets at all. A bone marrow biopsy differentiates between the destruction of platelets in the circulation or diminished production in the bone marrow. Thrombocytopenia requires treatment with corticosteroids or immunosuppressive agents. Increased destruction occurs in the spleen and results in splenomegaly. If drugs fail, a splenectomy will raise the platelet count. Surgical skills make laparoscopic splenectomy safe and easy. Before splenectomy, a pneumococcal vaccination should be given and then repeated every five years. Patients without spleens are at an increased risk for pneumococcal infections.

The white blood cell (WBC) count may be reduced in lupus patients. Low WBCs (leukopenia) increase susceptibility to infection. Granulocyte-stimulating factor (GSF) stimulates the production of the white cells. The commercial forms of GSF include Neupogen or Leukine. Unusual opportunistic infections occur as a consequence of leukopenia. On occasion, some lupus patients require prophylactic antibiotics. Vaccinations to prevent infection are encouraged.

Nephritis is a serious consequence of lupus. There are few signs or symptoms. The course of nephritis is variable. Often, the only abnormality is discovered in the urine analysis. The lupus patient with more serious nephritis may develop kidney (renal) failure. The leakage of protein into the urine (nephrotic syndrome) results in fluid retention, weight gain, edema, and ankle swelling. It is estimated that about one-third of patients with lupus will develop nephritis, which requires medical evaluation and treatment. A kidney biopsy is required to determine the prognosis and necessary treatment for nephritis. Despite treatment, some patients with lupus still go on to develop renal failure. Renal failure requires hemodialysis or peritoneal dialysis at home. Kidney transplantation has been successful in lupus patients with renal failure and eliminates the need for long-term dialysis. Kidney infection or hypertension also occurs. NSAIDs aggravate kidney function and hypertension. Appropriate medication prevents hypertension.

Criteria to Diagnose Lupus
◊   photosensitive skin rash
◊   facial rash in the malar distribution (butterfly rash)
◊   discoid rash
◊   painless mouth or nasal ulcers
◊   evidence of serositis
◊   abnormal urine analysis like protein, RBCs, or casts
◊   low blood counts
◊   neuropsychiatry problems
◊   positive ANA
◊   laboratory evidence of autoimmunity
◊   arthritis

Drug-Induced Lupus

Drug-induced lupus occurs after the use of some prescribed drugs in a small number of people. The symptoms of drug-induced lupus are similar to those of systemic lupus. A large percentage of the patients who take these drugs will develop antibodies suggestive of lupus, but only a small number will develop drug-induced lupus. The symptoms resolve when the medications are discontinued. Many of these medications are rarely used.

Pregnancy and Lupus

Lupus families have significant concern about pregnancy. Pregnancy poses unique and special problems for women with lupus. Even so, there are few reasons why a woman with lupus should not get pregnant. However, if involvement is active in organs like the central nervous system, kidney, heart, and lungs, the mother and fetus are at risk, and pregnancy is deferred. There is some risk of increased lupus activity during or immediately after pregnancy. Women with inactive lupus at the time of conception are less likely to experience a flare during pregnancy. If a person is monitored carefully during pregnancy, the dangers are minimized. For a woman with lupus who desires children, the timing of pregnancy is important. It is best if the mother is off most medicine and the lupus is determined to be inactive. Today, some lupus medications are being continued throughout pregnancy with careful monitoring. Fertility is normal in lupus, not only when the illness is quiescent, but also during periods of disease activity.

Pregnant lupus patients can develop the antiphospholipid syndrome. Antiphospholipid antibodies are responsible for some of the problems a pregnant lupus patient experiences while carrying a fetus to full term. Pregnant women with lupus have more stillbirths, premature deliveries, smaller birth weights, and miscarriages than individuals without lupus. During the antiphospholipid syndrome, there is a tendency to develop blood clots. If this occurs in the placenta, it significantly affects the fetus and the outcome of the pregnancy. In those lupus patients with a history of recurrent fetal losses because of autoantibodies (anticardiolipin, lupus anticoagulant), anticoagulation during pregnancy is required.

Research suggests that antimalarials can be utilized during pregnancy to prevent lupus flares and may be beneficial to prevent the antiphospholipid syndrome. Low doses of corticosteroids are used safely during pregnancy. If the doctor advises against pregnancy or children are not wanted, it is important to practice effective birth control measures. Unplanned pregnancy can occur. The safest form of birth control for women with lupus is a diaphragm with contraceptive foam and condoms, but birth control pills are still used.

Aspirin therapy is preferred to NSAIDs. Aspirin should be stopped within a few weeks of delivery to avoid excess bleeding. If flares do occur, corticosteroids during pregnancy do not appear to have an adverse effect on the fetus. There is a small risk of aggravating hypertension and diabetes in the mother. Prophylactic corticosteroids are not given during pregnancy, but those patients on long-term corticosteroid will need extra doses at the time of delivery for stress. Immunosuppressants are avoided because of the adverse effects on the fetus. Azathioprine is considered generally safe. Cyclophosphamide and methotrexate are contraindicated in pregnancy. Anticoagulants like warfarin are associated with an increased incidence of fetal loss during pregnancy. Low molecular weight anticoagulants, like subcutaneous injections of heparin (Lovenox), have been used more recently than intravenous heparin. Intravenous immunoglobulin (IVIG) is often used during pregnancy. Pregnancy is a special challenge in those individuals with connective tissue diseases. In lupus, conception and delivery should be timed when the underlying disease and its manifestations are well controlled. There are only a few patients who should avoid pregnancy. Pregnancy should not be avoided, but planned.

Neonatal Lupus Syndrome (NLS)

Maternal antibodies of pregnant lupus patients cross the placenta during the neonatal lupus syndrome (NLS). The presence of the Ro antibodies (SS-A) in the mother predicts transient rashes and heart block in the newborn. Maternal Ro antibodies are not a reason to terminate pregnancy, but their presence helps prepare for complications during delivery. The fetus and baby should be monitored closely during pregnancy, at the time of delivery, and postpartum.

Discoid Lupus

Discoid lupus is a variant of lupus that is limited to the skin. It occurs in about 10 percent of people with lupus. A characteristic rash appears on the face, neck, and scalp. The biopsy of the rash helps make the diagnosis. Discoid lupus does not involve the body's internal organs. It is not systemic. The ANA is usually negative in patients with discoid lupus. In a large number of patients with discoid lupus, the ANA test is positive, but at a low level. Only a small percentage of discoid lupus evolves into the systemic form of the disease. Treatment of discoid lupus will not prevent its progression to the systemic form. Individuals who progress to the systemic form probably had systemic lupus at the outset, with the discoid rash as their primary symptom complex. Lupus presents differently in all individuals. It is difficult to make comparisons from one person's illness to another. When people mention lupus, they are usually referring to the systemic form of the disease.

Mixed Connective Tissue Disease

Mixed connective tissue disease (MCTD) was originally described as a syndrome with a combination of features typical of patients with systemic lupus erythematosis, systemic sclerosis, polymyositis/dermatomyositis, or rheumatoid arthritis. A speckle-patterned ANA differentiates MCTD from other connective tissue diseases. Autoantibodies, like ribonucleoprotein (RNP) characterize MCTD. It has been a matter of controversy whether MCTD should be considered as a distinct entity. Some patients with MCTD develop clinical symptoms compatible with the pres-

ence of a well-defined connective tissue disease (CTD). Originally, MCTD was defined as a relatively benign disorder, but now it has been associated with significant organ involvement similar to other serious CTDs. The autoantibody RNP first described in MCTD has now been seen in other CTDs. The overlap of the laboratory findings has lead some experts to suggest MCTD be referred to as undifferentiated CTD or an overlap syndrome.

Treatment of Lupus

Preventive measures reduce the risk of lupus flares. Photosensitive patients must avoid excessive sun exposure and use the regular application of sunscreens to prevent rashes. Regular exercise helps prevent muscle weakness and fatigue. Immunization protects against specific infections. Estrogen replacement, weight-bearing exercise, calcium, and vitamin D supplements in postmenopausal women preserve bone density and minimize osteoporosis and risk for bone fracture. Support groups help alleviate the effects of stress. Treatment approaches are based on symptoms and laboratory findings. For the vast majority of people with lupus, effective treatment can minimize symptoms, reduce inflammation, and maintain normal functions. The course of lupus varies among people. Medications are prescribed depending on the organ system involved and the severity of the problem. Therapeutic options for patients with mild to moderate active lupus are usually limited to NSAIDs, antimalarials, and corticosteroids. Most often these medications manage the disease. In some patients, the management is incomplete and patients continue to have underlying inflammatory disease. In these situations, it is necessary to initiate immunosuppressive agents or large doses of corticosteroids. Unfortunately, large doses of corticosteroids are associated with guaranteed side effects.

Dehydroepiandrosterone (DHEA, prasterone) is a naturally occurring steroid produced by the adrenal glands. Early reports of lupus patients receiving 200 milligrams per day have demonstrated improvement. Improvement includes the reduction of corticosteroid doses and the associated side effects. Common adverse effects of prasterone include acne and extra hair growth, which is generally mild and treatable. However, DHEA is not intended to replace steroids, which are traditionally necessary to treat acute flares of lupus.

Cyclophosphamide (Cytoxan) is a potent immunosuppressant that historically has been given for cancer. Intravenous infusions are given monthly for six months for lupus nephritis, followed by doses at three monthly intervals. Other treatment includes pulse corticosteroids followed by oral corticosteroids and azathioprine (Imuran), another immunosuppressant. The response is significant and sustained. Mycophenolate mofetil (Cellcept) may be as beneficial as cyclophosphamide and safer in the management of nephritis.

New Drug Therapies

Rituximab (Rituxan) is an intravenous therapeutic investigational antibody that has shown an early favorable response in lupus and rheumatoid arthritis. This antibody specifically targets the CD20 antigen on the surface of some white cells (B-lymphocytes), which play an important role during the immune response and the inflammation of lupus. CD20 B-lymphocyte cells are attacked and killed by the rituximab. Stem cells and other B-lymphocytes do not all have the CD20 antigen on their cell surface. Rituximab has no effect on those cells without CD20 antigen on their cell surface. Therefore, the immune response is still preserved. Recent studies are evaluating rituximab's role as a first line therapy. Rituximab has already been approved in other conditions like relapsed or refractory non-Hodgkin's lymphoma and rheumatoid arthritis. Rituxan was the first therapeutic antibody approved for treating cancer in the United States. As we learn about this drug therapy and others, there is a growing body of experimental evidence that Rituxan and other biological agents will be able to deplete some B-lymphocytes that play a role in lupus. The favorable trend of clinical improvement and remarkable safety profile will encourage further research in this area. Intravenous infusions of rituximab appear to be safe and relatively easy to administer.

Prognosis of Lupus

The idea that lupus is generally a fatal disease is a misconception. The prognosis of lupus is better today than ever before. With early diagnosis and new and changing methods of therapy, including the judicious use of corticosteroids, 90 percent of people with lupus can look forward to a normal life span. Prior to current medical advances, most patient deaths were the result of kidney failure or involvement of the central nervous system. Today, as many patients with lupus will die from infection as from active disease. Lupus patients are more susceptible to infection because of the effects of lupus, or the treatment of lupus, on their immune status. These effects reduce their ability to prevent or fight infection and make them at risk for more infection and unusual infections (opportunistic). Many medications suppress the immune response and leave the patient more prone to infection. Although some people with lupus have severe recurrent flares and are frequently hospitalized, most people with lupus rarely require hospitalization. There are many lupus patients who have never been hospitalized.

CHAPTER FIVE

Fibromyalgia

Fibromyalgia (FM) is a common rheumatic disorder that affects an estimated 2 percent of the American population. It is more prevalent in women than in men. It is also known as soft-tissue rheumatism, fibrositis, non-articular rheumatism, or myofascial pain syndrome. Widespread aches and pains, fatigue, and poor sleep characterize fibromyalgia. Fibromyalgia is one of the most common problems for which people seek the advice of a physician. Arthritis sufferers also have fibromyalgia, yet fibromyalgia is really not a form of arthritis and will not harm the joints. A wealth of information has been learned about fibromyalgia. The cause of fibromyalgia has not been defined, but there are associations between the syndrome, physical injury, and psychological distress. Depending on physician training, fibromyalgia patients are seen by many different specialists.

Symptoms of Fibromyalgia

There are three important elements to fibromyalgia in the presence of overwhelming fatigue. There is a sleep disturbance. Individuals do not get deep sleep or stage-four sleep. They toss and turn. They are fitful sleepers. They get up at night with pain or discomfort and rather than fall back asleep quickly, they stay awake or get out of bed. Upon awakening, they are not rested. Later, during the day, they have difficulty coping with other problems. Sleep disturbance need not be the first symptom, but it occurs in conjunction with the other symptoms of fibromyalgia. Fibromyalgia has long been linked to psychological disturbance. The patients are depressed, discouraged, or distressed. They don't always see the light at the end of the tunnel. They are fatigued and lack energy or endurance. Characteristic tender points have been mapped out. Trigger points occur at the base of the skull, neck and shoulders, elbows, low back, breastbone, hips, or the knees. These areas are extremely painful to touch. The pain is very real. If you take a scalpel and cut across these areas, nothing is found, even under the microscope. When these areas are touched or palpated, the patient response is usually abrupt withdrawal, out of proportion to the pressure applied. The doctor may not be aware of these areas until the patient is examined.

Fibromyalgia is a collection of symptoms without a definitive test to define it. It quickly becomes a vicious cycle. The cycle easily escalates and snowballs. There may be a precipitating event, like a back injury, car accident, or fall. Fibromyalgia can be disabling. If symptoms occur for a short while, the prognosis is much better than if the symptoms are ongoing for a long period of time. At the time of diagnosis, most people have many years of symptoms. There is no routine laboratory test, x-ray, or other procedure of diagnostic or prognostic value in fibromyalgia.

The American College of Rheumatology has established criteria to identify fibromyalgia. These criteria appear to be relatively simple, sensitive, and specific. Some critics suggest that individuals should not be mislabeled with this diagnosis. Unfortunately, many people are subjected to unnecessary diagnostic tests, and in some cases surgery, before the diagnosis is well established. Establishing the label early prevents unnecessary testing and procedures. Fulfilling all

the criteria established by the ACR is not always necessary, unless one is carrying out a clinical trial where it is important that all the patients meet the same criteria. Headache, irritable bowel syndrome, chronic fatigue, temperomandibular pain, and mood disorders can all be part of fibromyalgia.

Criteria to Establish Fibromyalgia

◊ widespread pain for on both right and left sides of the body
◊ pressure applied to at least eleven out of eighteen trigger points

---

Treatment of Fibromyalgia

Surgery for fibromyalgia should be avoided and narcotics kept to a minimum. The lack of understanding of the basis of the disease and lower pain levels results in therapy being empiric. Pain cannot be cut out. Unfortunately, many of these individuals are subjected to surgeries in an attempt to rid them of pain. Narcotics do not get at the source of the problem. Many times, narcotics provide an opportunity for abuse, dependence, and even addiction. Early treatment should be nonpharmacological and include counseling, exercise, and education.

Trigger Points of Fibromyalgia

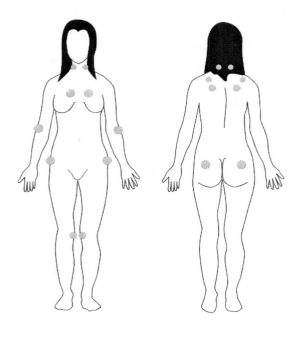

When these methods fail, antidepressant medications at night are helpful. Antidepressants help with sleep, improve mood, and elevate the brain's threshold for pain without creating dependency on medication. Any intervention that breaks the cycle of pain, poor sleep, and depression will be of benefit. Local steroid injections, massage, or physical therapy are helpful and have little risk.

Individuals seek alternative treatment providers including the chiropractor, massage therapist, or acupuncturist. All will be helpful to some degree. Exercise, behavioral therapy, and many alternative treatments have the potential to change the way the brain interprets pain and ultimately pain levels. Teaching patients the benefits of relaxation therapy, visual imagery, and coping skills are all helpful. Problem solving and goal setting reduce pain and allow patients a sense of well being and control of their pain response. Coping strategies develop a sense of a control and influences how the brain reacts to pain.

The tricyclic antidepressant medications are the most extensively studied adjunctive medications in pain management. They have proven efficacy. Their primary mechanism of action is believed to occur by inhibition of norepinephrine and serotonin reuptake, both of which are important neurotransmitters of pain. Common side effects include dry mouth, urinary retention, visual changes, and sedation. They are contraindicated in people with glaucoma and a history of urinary retention.

Tricyclic antidepressants like amitriptyline (Elavil) and muscle relaxants like cyclobenzaprine (Flexeril) are effective in the short-term treatment of fibromyalgia and have been available in the United States for over thirty years. With these agents, most people will have a modest degree of improvement. Some will have dramatic improvement of symptoms. It is impossible to identify those who will respond. Medication doses are usually lower than what would be expected to modify mood. Since the side effects of antidepressants are mild and resolve quickly with discontinuation of medication, drug treatment is often warranted. Small doses of amitriptyline are taken at bedtime to help sleep and earlier in the evening if there is morning-after sedation. Side effects like dry mouth or excessive sedation improve with time. Other side effects of tricyclic antidepressants like weight gain, nightmares, constipation, dreaming, and occasional paradoxical insomnia are usually unacceptable. Antidepressants are continued for several months and then tapered or discontinued. About 40 percent of patients achieve a useful clinical response over a few weeks. In some situations, antidepressants are continued for years. The generic antidepressant drugs are relatively inexpensive. An antidepressant is given in conjunction with other management strategies after a careful discussion about the course and prognosis of fibromyalgia. Tricyclic antidepressants relieve pain regardless of whether patients are depressed. Desipramine (Norpramine) has the best side effect profile of all the tricyclic antidepressants.

Because the tricyclics have numerous side effects and are frequently poorly tolerated by patients, the newer selective serotonin reuptake inhibitor (SSRI) class of antidepressants has been studied. Their relative selectivity has resulted in less promising results than the tricyclics.

It is unclear whether antidepressants that are SSRIs like fluoxetine (Prozac), paroxetine (Paxil), sertraline (Zoloft), citalopram (Celexa), or escitalpram (Lexapro) are of more value than traditional tricyclic antidepressants. More people discontinue treatment with tricyclic antidepressants because of side effects than do people taking SSRIs. On occasion SSRIs are used in conjunction with the antidepressants like amitriptyline. Drug interactions can result in excess blood levels. Drug interaction with tricyclics is not problematic with citalopram and escitalopram.

Anti-anxiety medications are of limited value. Early enthusiasm for them has been tempered by the concern for dependence and possible withdrawal symptoms. Anti-inflammatory medications, except for their mild effect on pain, appear to have little if any value in the treatment of fibromyalgia.

Finally, an ingredient of cough syrup readily available is guaifenesin. Its use in FM is controversial.

Individuals with fibromyalgia often fall prey to unproven remedies or unconventional treatment programs. Unproven remedies do not do any direct harm, but raise false hope and cause disappointment when there is no relief, lighten the pocketbook, and keep patients away from conventional medical care delaying the diagnosis.

Local injection of tender points with corticosteroid and an anesthetic are utilized with some success. Injections should be limited in number. Chiropractic manipulation and myofascial therapy (spray and stretch) have had limited success. Topical lidocaine patches (5 percent Lidoderm patches) are FDA-approved for the pain of postherpetic neuralgia secondary to shingles and have been used in a variety of other localized areas of pain. The patches are worn until they will no longer stick to the skin. The patches are cut to size and useful for small, localized areas of pain. The patches in combination with an oral medication for sleep disorders like modafinil (Provigil) are useful. Provigil promotes wakefulness.

Most skeletal muscle relaxants like diazepam (Valium), lorazepam (Ativan), clonazepam (Klonopin), other sedatives, or even antihistamines carry the risk of dependence. Carisoprodol (Soma) is a commonly used muscle relaxant that can cause dependence. If used for long periods, patients often have difficulty discontinuing the medication. Gabapentin (Neurontin), normally an anti-seizure drug, is useful for chronic pain syndromes and is given three times daily to be effective. Neurontin is well tolerated; however, treatment for pain is considered off-label use. A similar drug, pregabalin (Lyrica), is also available and is used in an off-label fashion like gabapentin. Dosing is twice a day. Otherwise, pregabalin is approved for painful diabetic neuropathy and postherpetic neuralgia. Education and exercise are important ingredients and adjuvants of any treatment program for the fibromyalgia patient.

Dually focused treatment of fibromyalgia includes the combination of drug and nondrug therapies.

Spectrum of Fibromyalgia

The temporomandibular joint disorder (TMJ) is often involved in fibromyalgia. More than a third of fibromyalgia patients have jaw pain at the temporomandibular joint. This condition is more common in women, as is fibromyalgia. For many people, these two disorders and their symptoms overlap. Jaw pain easily affects the muscles of the face, head, neck, shoulder, and back. Other symptoms include tenderness chewing, locking of the joint, and teeth grinding. There is no value of surgery for the overwhelming majority of people with TMJ disorder. Adjusting the alignment of the teeth and improving the bite can be helpful. Splints, orthodontics, stress reduction can all be helpful. The key to treatment must include non-invasive approaches until they clearly fail. Pain in the area of hip bursa or tennis elbow will sometimes be part of fibromyalgia, too.

There is an overlap between fibromyalgia and chronic fatigue syndrome (CFS). Similarities suggest that these two syndromes are possibly at different ends of the same spectrum of disease. Chronic fatigue syndrome is defined by severe fatigue of at least six months duration that interferes substantially with usual activities of living. It has no characteristic physical signs or accompanying laboratory abnormalities and poses a diagnostic and management challenge. Despite the protracted chronic nature of CFS and the severity of associated impairment and disability, CFS is still not adequately recognized or managed. This reflects lack of access to health care or inadequate knowledge by those providing services.

Hope Is Here

Fibromyalgia should not be interpreted as a disabling or crippling condition, but rather as a chronic disorder with available effective therapies. There is no cure. Patients must take an active role in their treatment as compared to a passive role. Patient support groups are helpful. Fibromyalgia is a disorder of exclusion. It is important to ensure other illnesses are not present that could explain the symptoms. Hypothyroidism or other more serious disease can be confused with the symptoms of fibromyalgia. Fibromyalgia occurs more frequently with other rheumatic illnesses, including rheumatoid arthritis. Other serious illnesses are associated with mood changes, poor sleep, and pain. An examination by a medical doctor sorts out many of these other problems. New drugs will potentially help patients with the burden of fibromyalgia, but they need to be added cautiously to other selected nonpharmacological management strategies. Although research has looked for an immunological basis for fibromyalgia and found many unusual

laboratory abnormalities in these patients, no definite relationship has been established.

CHAPTER SIX

Gout

Gout is a disease that has been studied since antiquity. Gout was thought to be a disease of the affluent and primarily observed in middle-aged men of the wealthy upper class. It was described as a disease of kings and king of disease, due to its association with rich food and alcohol consumption. Colorful depictions of gout are found in art and literature, often with commentary on the moral character of the gout sufferer. During these times, gout has kept good company, afflicting King Alexander the Great, Henry VIII, Benjamin Franklin, Alexander Hamilton, Charles Darwin, and Leonardo da Vinci. Gout was associated with the wealthy, educated, and those individuals who could afford the excesses of life. Their habits included overindulgence, gluttony, and lack of willpower. Chronic lead intoxication as a result of contamination during homemade winemaking explained some historic epidemics of gout during the Roman Empire. Lead toxicity impairs the ability of the kidney to excrete uric acid. It is now postulated that diet has a greater effect on gout than does alcohol.

Gout is characterized by an acute and recurrent monoarthritis arthritis created by the crystallization of uric acid within the joint and is typically associated with a high serum uric acid level. Once inside the joint, the crystal precipitates a sudden and intense inflammatory response that results in an acute swelling, redness, warmth, and pain of the joint. Since uric acid concentrations fluctuate, the uric acid measurement during an acute attack is not diagnostic and rarely useful. The uric acid level may be low or high during the time of an attack.

Gout is a common medical problem that affects at least 1 percent of adult men in America. Acute attacks are episodic. Men get the first attack of gout at about the third decade of life. Unless there is a rare inherited problem with metabolism, it is unusual to get gout any younger. Women get gout after menopause. Gout is recognized as the most common form of acute arthritis in males over forty years of age. In the industrialized countries, there appears to be an increasing prevalence and presentation earlier in life. Excessive alcohol intake, hypertension, diuretic drug therapy, and obesity contribute to the risk of developing gout and elevated uric acid levels. Consumption of red meat and seafood, and decreased consumption of dairy products also contributes to the increasing prevalence of gout. The declining use of hormone replacement therapy in postmenopausal women may increase the incidence of gout. Gout is increasing in urban communities and populations that historically were not bothered by gout. Gout is no longer the disease of the wealthy; rather, its appearance reflects Western civilization diets of excess. Gout is consistent with poor dietary trends in America.

Uric acid concentrations are monitored over several weeks to determine if they are elevated, not only at the time of an attack. Changes of the uric acid level up or down are often responsible for precipitating an acute attack. A low uric measurement does not exclude the diagnosis of gout and neither does an elevated uric acid level confirm gout. Demonstrating a single uric acid crystal in the joint fluid is required to make the diagnosis. The presentation may be classical enough that gout can be highly suspected at the bedside or clinic. The blood uric acid level is still the most important determinant of the risk for developing gout.

Clinical Course of Gout

The first attack of gout usually involves the big toe—75 percent of the time. Gout in this location is referred to as podagra. During the course of gout, attacks occur in the big toe 95 percent of the time. Other lower extremity joints, including the knee, ankle, or foot, are at risk for acute attacks. Polyarticular gout is characterized by acute attacks occurring in several joints at the same time. Individuals seek out urgent medical attention because attacks are so painful. The inflammation is acute and can cause systemic symptoms like fever. The attack and inflammation mimics infection. The treatment to suppress the inflammation is very different from the treatment to decrease the uric acid levels. Untreated, gout lasts several days and then resolves on its own. Until it resolves, the discomfort is severe. Gout is often frequent and recurrent. Subsequent attacks occur more often and are more frequent. Treatment results in relief in a matter of hours, with complete resolution in a few days.

Gout occurs in three overlapping stages. The stages include a long phase of asymptomatic elevated uric acid levels, a period of recurrent acute gouty attacks of sudden onset, separated by asymptomatic intervals or periods without symptoms, followed by chronic tophaceous gouty arthritis in about 10 percent of patients. Tophi are large collections of uric acid crystals deposited in the connective tissues outside the joints. Tophi are common in patients with untreated or inadequately treated elevated uric acid levels and develop over many years.

Treatment of an Acute Attack

An acute attack requires a drug treatment program different from the medications used to lower the elevated uric acid. Treatment is first directed against the acute inflammation. Nonsteroidal anti-inflammatories (NSAIDs) are helpful and should be started at the first sign of inflammation. Patients with recurrent gout attacks usually recognize the signs and symptoms early and can abort full-blown gout attacks with oral NSAIDs. Indomethacin (Indocin/Indocin SR) has been a favorite NSAID, but most all NSAIDs are helpful, including the selective COX-2 agents. Early, high doses of NSAIDs followed by tapering doses bring rapid relief. On occasion, it is necessary to use oral corticosteroids or even intra-articular corticosteroids. Corticosteroids by any route work well and quickly. The drug colchicine has also been used for many years in acute attacks of gout. Colchicine often causes gastrointestinal symptoms of nausea, vomiting, cramps, or diarrhea in large doses. After the initial doses of colchicine, relief begins quickly, but

so may the gastrointestinal symptoms. Colchicine works dramatically for the acute inflammation, but it is difficult to know which is worse, the gastrointestinal symptoms of the colchicine or the gout attack. If fewer than two tablets are used daily, colchicine is well tolerated and still effective. Colchicine is given for a few months to prevent future attacks of gout. It is amazing how effective this small birdseed-sized colchicine pill (0.6 milligrams) is for gout.

Treating the Uric Acid Problem

Elevated serum uric acid levels occur at some time or another, before attacks occur. Either too much uric acid is produced by the body or too little is excreted by the kidneys. The end result is hyperuricemia. Hyperuricemia may or may not be associated with actual gout attacks. If the uric acid level is severely elevated or associated with multiple gout attacks, it is necessary to treat the elevated uric acid concentrations with the drug allopurinol (Zyloprim). Allopurinol is a xanthine oxidase inhibitor and inhibits the production of uric acid. The drug probenecid (Benemid) increases the excretion of uric acid in the urine and is also effective. Increasing the amount of uric acid in the urine is not desirable if kidney stones have been a problem.

Fuboxostat is an emerging drug and will be a potential new gout treatment approved by the FDA soon. There has been no new gout treatment for the past forty years. Favorable, early studies suggest febuxostat (Uloric) lowers uric acid well. Since all patients cannot tolerate allopurinol, this drug may provide a potent useful alternative. Fenofibrate (Tricor), a lipid-lowering agent, and losartan (Cozaar), a high blood pressure medication, can modestly reduce uric acid and may be useful in combination with allopurinol in those patients that have elevated lipids or high blood pressure.

Prevention of Gout

The prevention of gouty arthritis in the asymptomatic phase consists of the correction of secondary causes of hyperuricemia, including eliminating drugs like diuretics low-dose aspirin, avoiding laxative abuse, limiting consumption of alcoholic, gradual weight reduction for obese patients, and dietary restriction of purine-rich foods. Foods rich in purines include shellfish and organ meats like brain, heart, and kidney. These measures constitute sufficient therapy for many patients. Gout patients are often overweight, and their blood pressure is often elevated. Some diuretic drug therapies for elevated blood pressure like thiazides (Dyazide, Hydrodiuril) or furosemide (Lasix) worsen and increase uric acid concentrations. They are best avoided if possible. Other blood pressure medications will not aggravate uric acid concentrations.

The prevention of gouty attacks depends on normalization of the serum uric acid concentration. The frequency and severity of attacks can be reduced by the prophylactic administration of small doses of 0.6 milligram colchicine tablets once or twice daily. Larger doses of colchicine are avoided because of intolerance and gastrointestinal side effects like cramps, nausea, and diarrhea. Chronic colchicine treatment does not reverse hyperuricemia and does nothing to prevent asymptomatic and progressive tophaceous disease. There is no doubt that patients with sustained significant hyperuricemia who experience frequent gouty attacks of more than four a year require long-term treatment with drugs to lower uric levels.

Diet

Gout is often called the disease of the wealthy because of the potential contribution of rich foods to the cause. It is better called the "disease of plenty." During medieval times, individuals feasted and often developed gout. This resulted in the belief that rich foods contribute to the cause of gout. Today, few people eat foods rich in purines like brain, liver, sweetbreads, or other organ meats on a regular basis. Other foods high in purines include oily fish, seafood, beans, peas, oatmeal, spinach, asparagus, cauliflower, and mushrooms. Dietary efforts are usually not totally effective in controlling gout. Serum uric acid levels are determined not only by the purine content of food, but also by the rate at which the kidneys eliminate the uric acid and by additional purine formation that occurs in the body. In reality, food contributes only a small portion of the excess uric acid present in gout patients. Restriction of purine-containing foods is of some benefit; however, medications are far more effective.

The recent popularity of low carbohydrate diets may have a deleterious effect on uric acid levels and the incidence of gout, but this currently remains to be determined. Moderate wine consumption is not associated with a risk of developing gout, but regular moderate consumption of beer is associated with a significant risk. All alcohol consumption should be kept to the minimum. Recent studies have suggested, but not definitely established, that the regular consumption of dairy products may diminish the risk of gout and actually lower uric acid levels.

Dietary trends are contributing to the increasing prevalence of gout, obesity, and the metabolic syndrome in the United States. Gout patients need to pay attention to weight management. Weight management has the potential to lower serum uric acid levels.

Anecdotally, cherries are the number one home dietary remedy for gout. No studies have been conducted to confirm how cherries work; people suspect that cherries contain an enzyme that helps break down and promote the excretion of uric acid. This remains to be proven. Consumption of black cherry juice can-

not be universally recommended as a remedy for gout at this time.

Colchicine

Colchicine, a drug derived from the roots of the autumn crocus *(Colchium autumnale),* is one of the oldest remedies for gout. There are three indications for the use of colchicine in the treatment of gout.

Indications for Colchicine
◊   a supplement to anti-inflammatories for acute gout ◊   prophylaxis prior to an acute attack ◊   prophylaxis when initiating uric acid-lowering agents

Once considered the mainstay in the treatment of acute gout, colchicine is now used infrequently because of its adverse effects. Colchicine is more effective when used early, especially during the first twenty-four hours of onset of an acute gout attack. All too often, patients do not start taking colchicine until a day or so following the onset of an attack. Oral colchicine is useful in two-thirds of patients presenting with acute gout. Many people experience nausea, vomiting, diarrhea, and abdominal pain before full improvement. This narrow benefit-to-toxicity ratio has limited the use of colchicine. Corticosteroids and NSAIDs

Criteria for the Diagnosis of Gout
◊   more than one attack of acute arthritis
◊   maximum inflammation of the joint developed within one day
◊   arthritis attack in only one joint
◊   severe redness observed over joints
◊   great toe painful, swollen, and red
◊   first attack of one great toe
◊   midfoot joint attack of one side only
◊   collections of uric acid crystals (tophi)
◊   elevated uric acid levels demonstrated
◊   characteristic joint changes on x-ray
◊   characteristic crystals demonstrated in joint fluid

are better tolerated, more efficacious, and are the first choice of most rheumatologists in the treatment of acute gout.

Advice about Acute Attacks

An attack of acute gout away from home is difficult. The rapid and early institution of either colchicine or an anti-inflammatory helps quickly. Occasionally, attacks are resistant to traditional medications, so that either injectable or oral corticosteroids are utilized. Oral corticosteroids like methylprednisolone (Medrol Dosepack) are useful. The initial dose is tapered slowly over a few days. Extended use of corticosteroids is usually avoided. Acute attacks of gout, regardless of the location, including the joint, bursa, or tendon, are extremely painful. The pain of acute attacks compares to having surgery without anesthesia. Gout patients in our arthritis clinic are the only patients to come to the clinic with one shoe on and the other off, on axillary crutches, or with a portion of their tennis shoe cut out to take pressure off a painful big toe. Treatment responds to anti-inflammatories so well that analgesics are rarely needed. Gout is one of the most painful rheumatic diseases, but one of the most gratifying to treat.

Tophaceous Gout

There are few reasons for chronic tophaceous gout in modern times. Individuals allergic to the medicine, or who do not comply with taking their medicine, have difficulty lowering their uric acid concentrations and develop tophi over many years. Tophi are uric acid collections easily visible on the fingers, elbows, or even the ears. The examination of a tophus under a polarizing microscope reveals thousands of negatively birefringent crystals. A tophus is characterized by a lack of inflammatory cells. Typically, tophi erode the bone and can easily be seen on a radiograph of the hands or feet. Magnetic resonance imaging demonstrates soft tissue collections of tophi. Tophi are pea or grapefruit sized. Material expressed from tophi is a cheesy white paste that contains thousands of microscopic uric acid crystals. Allopurinol is the treatment of choice for tophaceous gout and is continued indefinitely. Allopurinol is not started during an acute attack. Concurrent administration of colchicine prevents attacks at the time of initiation of allopurinol, as the uric acid level is quickly decreased. Noncompliance in patients with tophaceous gout will lead to one acute attack after another.

Drugs Useful in the Treatment of Gout

- ◇ Allopurinol lowers the uric acid.
- ◇ Probenecid lowers the uric acid.
- ◇ Colchicine is more prophylactic than useful acutely.
- ◇ NSAIDs help the acute inflammation of gout.
- ◇ Steroids are the most powerful anti-inflammatory.

Pseudogout

Pseudogout is an acute self-limiting arthritis similar to the acute inflammation of gout. Regardless of treatment, the arthritis usually resolves on its own. It is predominately a disease of the elderly and targets the knees, wrists, shoulders, and hips. Acute episodes are caused by the body's reaction to crystalline deposits within the joint and cartilage. The difference between pseudogout and gout are the crystals and the specific joints affected. The chronic form of pseudogout has a strong association with osteoarthritis and some endocrine abnormalities. Intra-articular calcification deposition of calcium pyrophosphate dihydrate (CPPD) crystals is seen faintly on x-rays (chondrocalcinosis).

There is a preponderance of female patients and a striking association with aging. Chondrocalcinosis is most unusual in persons under the age of fifty. Numerous metabolic diseases occur concurrently including diabetes, Paget's disease, thyroid disease, hemachromatosis, and hyperparathyroidism. Pseudogout is the most common cause of acute monoarthritis in the elderly. Acute arthritis of pseudogout is the only symptom of asymptomatic calcification of cartilage seen on x-ray. The cartilage of the joint becomes saturated with calcium crystals. It is unclear why the calcium is shed from the cartilage. The knees are the most common joints involved. A typical attack occurs rapidly and without warning. The attack is characterized by severe pain and inflammation. The joint is swollen, red, warm, and painful. Attacks usually resolve over several days. Most attacks occur spontaneously.

In chronic forms of pseudogout, symptoms are often restricted to a few joints (oligoarthritis), although mono-articular and polyarticular forms occur too. Polyarticular pseudogout mimics rheumatoid arthritis. Attacks are super-imposed on chronic pain, stiffness, and limitation of movement because of OA. Severe destructive arthritis occurs on occasion. Osteoarthritis is a common ac-companiment. Involvement of the knee often results in fixed flexion deformities of the joint and makes ambulation diffi-cult. During acute attacks, pillows under the knees provide comfort, but their use should be avoided to prevent flexion de-formities.

Five Presentations of Pseudogout

◊ attacks in one joint like gout
◊ pseudo-rheumatoid arthritis
◊ progressive joint degradation
◊ x-ray calcification with disease
◊ chronic destructive arthropathy, especially the shoulder

A destructive arthropathy is not unusual. The Milwaukee shoulder is a syndrome that classically affects the el-derly patient with long-standing shoul-der pain complicated by a large degree of swelling. Removal of the fluid from a swollen joint provides an opportunity to demonstrate calcium pyrophosphate crystals. The crystal is characteristically different from the crystal of gout. The crystals of CPPD are faintly positive bi-refringent when visualized under a polar-izing microscope. Even with a polarizing microscope, the crystal is difficult to see. Calcification of cartilage is seen faintly on x-rays, especially in the fibrocartilage of the knee or wrists, but also in hyaline cartilage of the knee, shoulder, or hip.

The goal of medical management is to reduce the painful symptoms quickly, to identify and verify the cause as pseu-dogout, and to mobilize the patient as early as possible. Simple oral analgesics and most NSAIDs give relief. Colchi-cine is rarely used. Intra-articular or oral corticosteroids are necessary on occasion. Unlike gout, pseudogout has no specific therapy. Treatment of any underlying metabolic disease does not necessarily influence outcome. Avoid-ance of foods in the diet has no effect on pseudogout. On occasion, pseudogout is a chronic condition.

CHAPTER SEVEN

Spondyloarthropathies

Ankylosing spondylitis, psoriatic arthritis, Reiter's syndrome, and the arthritis associated with inflammatory bowel disease like Crohn's disease and ulcerative colitis represent the seronegative spondyloarthropathies. All are more common in men and have a tendency to involve the spine. The rheumatoid factor is negative. Inflammation of the spine (spondyloarthropathy) begins in the sacroiliac joints and ascends up the spine over many years. There is no definite laboratory test to establish the diagnosis. The HLA B27 genetic marker occurs in more than 90 percent of the patients, but it is also present in 6 percent of the normal population. There is a tendency for inflammation at the tendon attachments to bone (enthesopathy). These areas calcify and are visible on x-ray. Excess calcification complicates joint replacement.

Ankylosing Spondylitis

Ankylosing spondylitis (AS) is a form of arthritis primarily affecting young men. Women develop the disease less often. Spinal involvement is usually the first manifestation. Inflammation of the spine develops slowly during the late teens and early twenties and ascends up the spine over many years. The first symptom is low backache. Many people mistakenly attribute these symptoms to excessive bending, lifting, sitting, or sleeping in an awkward position. Unlike most low back pain, the pain associated with AS is worse during periods of rest or inactivity. Patients do better with exercise.

Characteristic bone formations (syndesmophytes) join adjacent vertebras. Syndesmophytes are different from the osteophytes seen in OA. The inflammation stiffens the spine and results in loss of flexibility. Syndesmophytes are so extensive that the spine takes on a bamboo appearance on x-ray. Inflammation fuses the sacroiliac joints, which are the earliest area of involvement. The fusion of the sacroiliac joints is visualized by x-ray or by CT scanning. Over a long period of time, posture becomes stooped. Stooped posture is corrected by difficult and extensive spinal surgery. Peripheral arthritis of the joints occurs. Systemic symptoms include inflammation of the anterior portion of the eye (iritis), inflammation of the upper lung fields (confused with tuberculosis), and disturbances of the electrical conduction of the heart. The mainstay of treatment is NSAIDs, but biological anti-TNFs are being used more often.

Psoriasis Arthritis

Psoriasis is a noncontagious skin disorder that appears as an inflamed rash and skin lesions covered with silvery white scales. Psoriatic patches occur in many areas of the body but are more often found in the scalp, elbows, knees, and low back. Rash confined to the scalp must be sought carefully within the hairline. Patients are not always aware of their psoriasis and attribute a rash in their scalp to dandruff. Psoriasis commonly affects the nails and causes pitting, ridging, or lifting of the nails (onycholysis). The rash does not follow a predictable course.

Psoriatic arthritis (PsA) is a chronic inflammatory arthritis associated with psoriasis in the absence of a positive test for rheumatoid factor. Initially, psoriatic arthritis was considered a variant of rheumatoid arthritis, but it has now emerged as a distinct clinical entity. The swelling of the fingers or toes gives an appearance of sausage digits. Swelling is not only confined to the area of the finger joint; it involves the entire digit.

No one knows what causes psoriasis. Six million Americans are affected by psoriasis. Women and men are affected equally. The arthritis occurs in a small percentage of those people with the rash, but can occur before the rash is obvious. Activity of the arthritis correlates to the activity of the skin rash. Gout is more common in individuals with psoriasis. The laboratory tests and markers for other forms of rheumatic illness are negative. Psoriatic arthritis has several forms.

Forms of Psoriatic Arthritis
◊ symmetric polyarthritis like rheumatoid arthritis
◊ low back pain and involvement of the sacroiliac joints
◊ involvement limited to the distal interphalangeal joints of the fingers
◊ asymmetric involvement of less than five joints
◊ arthritis mutilans of the fingers, with rapid destruction of the joints

Treatment of Psoriatic Arthritis

Controlling the skin rash is essential to the treatment. Good skin care is important. Phototherapy is helpful. Many patients do better in the sunshine during the summer months. Systemic corticosteroids are typically avoided. Corticosteroids reduce the efficacy of other disease modifying antirheumatic drugs and on cessation lead to rebound. The response to oral corticosteroids is limited and leads to increasing doses. Oral corticosteroids complicate the disease. Topical corticosteroids applied to the skin are useful for the skin rash, but not for the arthritis. Mild arthritis is controlled by oral anti-inflammatory medications. Just as with RA, DMARDs are instituted early in the course of PsA, particularly when the course resembles RA. The most commonly used oral agents are MTX (Trexall, Rheumatrex), sulfasalazine (Azulfidine), or hydroxychloroquine (Plaquenil). Methotrexate is the DMARD of choice because of its efficacy in both skin and joint disease. MTX can be used with other DMARDs, including biologicals. Gold injections have been used to treat the arthritis, but can aggravate the rash.

The anti-TNF medications have taken on an important role in the treatment of the arthritis and rash of psoriasis. These biological agents are used in the treatment of both the rash and arthritis and are well tolerated. Etanercept may be used as monotherapy without MTX. Infliximab is given concurrently with MTX. It is expected that other anti-TNF medications will be approved for the treatment of PsA.

Reiter's Syndrome

Reiter's syndrome is characterized by inflammation of the joints, eyes, and the genital, urinary, or gastrointestinal systems. Reiter's syndrome is a reactive arthritis. Inflammation is the result of the immune system's response to the presence of bacterial infection of the genital, urinary, or gastrointestinal systems. Typically, the arthritis develops a few weeks after the onset of the infection and involves the knees, ankles, feet, or wrists. Some causative agents include chlamydia, salmonella, yersinia, or shigella bacteria. Often, the source of infection is never found. The arthritis is usually asymmetrical. The rheumatoid factor is negative. In comparison to other forms of arthritis, fluid accumulation in the knee is extensive. Similar to other seronegative spondyloarthropathies, the inflammation of an entire finger or toe gives the appearance of a sausage digit. Inflammation at the insertion of the tendons results in tendinitis. Achilles tendinitis is common and causes swelling and heel pain. Inflammation of the eyes is usually confined to conjunctivitis and is not painful. If iritis occurs, it is painful and interferes with vision. Any portion of the urinary tract may be involved and entirely asymptomatic. Inflammation of the urinary tract is discovered by an abnormal urine analysis, painful urgency with urination, or urethral discharge. Painless sores of the mouth occur and go unnoticed. Inflammation of the large bowel precipitates diarrhea. Skin inflammation occurs on the penis or bottom of the feet. Less common areas of involvement include inflammation of the aortic valve or the electrical conduction pathway of the heart. The areas of involvement determine treatment.

Treatment of Reiter's Syndrome

Arthritis and other aspects of Reiter's syndrome will often resolve spontaneously within the first year. A number of patients will not require intervention. NSAIDs and intra-articular or oral corticosteroids provide relief. Topical steroid drops are used for the eye inflammation and corticosteroid creams for the rashes. Since iritis can result in blindness, the ophthalmologist will see affected individuals for further treatment. Treatment with antibiotics is not always necessary. Those individuals with chronic evidence of arthritis find DMARDs helpful. DMARDs are often used when the arthritis resembles RA.

Arthritis-Associated Inflammatory Bowel Disease

Inflammatory bowel disease (IBD) is a group of chronic disorders that results in ulceration of the small and large intestines. Ulcerative colitis and Crohn's disease are inflammatory bowel disorders. The inflammation of Crohn's extends into the deeper layers of the intestinal wall, while ulcerative colitis is more superficial. The inflammatory arthritis associated with IBD is characterized by remissions and exacerbations. Common symptoms include abdominal pain, diarrhea, rectal bleeding, weight loss, and fever. Arthritis occurs in a small percentage of patients. The arthritis occasionally precedes the bowel involvement, but usually coincides with the activity of the bowel disease. Lower extremity migratory arthritis is most common. Migratory arthritis moves from one joint to another in a short while, leaving the first joint without symptoms. The arthritis associated with IBD creates tremendous inflammation of the joint and is characterized by severe swelling of the joint space. The rheumatoid factor is negative. The arthritis usually lasts only a short time and does not cause permanent damage. Once the bowel symptoms are under control the outlook for the joints is excellent.

General Treatment Guidelines of Seronegative Spondyloarthropathy

The therapy and natural course of seronegative spondyloarthropathies have many things in common. Since patients do better with exercise, regular activity is promoted. Maintaining good posture is critical. Periods of rest and relaxation between activities are important. Maintaining erect posture avoids stooping later. Sleeping prone (face down) is preferred to sleeping supine, but is difficult for many people. Once a stooped posture begins, it becomes more difficult to correct. Pillows behind the knees encourage fixed flexion deformities and should be avoided. Since it is an aerobic exercise and improves flexibility and deep breathing, swimming is one of the best activities. Anti-inflammatories are frequently used. DMARDs are used in those individuals with a peripheral arthritis similar to RA. For those people undergoing major joint replacement, indomethacin (Indocin) is given to discourage extra bone formation or calcification around the new joint. The biologicals are playing an increasingly important role in treatment.

CHAPTER EIGHT

Scleroderma

Scleroderma is a collagen vascular disease characterized by the overproduction of collagen. There is involvement of the vascular, inflammatory, and fibrotic processes of the skin. Fibrosis is the hallmark of the disease. Progressive systemic sclerosis (PSS) is another term for scleroderma. Morphia is a localized form of scleroderma and results in a hard patch of involved skin that improves with time. Eosinophilic fasciitis is a variant of PSS. Although not entirely unique to PSS, color changes (Raynaud's phenomenon) of the fingers and hands, calcifications (calcinosis) just under the skin, swallowing difficulties (dysphasia), tightening of the skin (sclerodactyly) at the fingers, and dilated small blood vessels (telangectasia) under the skin, especially on the face, are common. Scleroderma literally means hard skin. The cause of scleroderma is unknown. It occurs most commonly in young and middle age women between the ages of twenty-five and thirty-five years of age, although men also develop PSS. If vital organ involvement occurs, the disease is life threatening, otherwise the course is variable and often mild. It is chronic and usually lasts a lifetime. Occasional spontaneous remissions occur. It is estimated that as many as one hundred thousand Americans have scleroderma. Even so, it is still an uncommon disease.

Excess collagen is deposited in the skin and other organs. Damage occurs to internal organs from the accumulation of collagen. Collagen is found in the tissues connecting muscles to bones, but also other connective tissues like skin, cartilage, and ligaments. Internal organs get stiff and function poorly. Small blood vessel involvement is a prominent part of scleroderma. Vascular and collagen involvement explains the term collagen vascular disease. Lung (interstitial fibrosis) or kidney (kidney failure or hypertension) involvement indicates a poor prognosis and encourages aggressive management.

Classical Symptoms of Scleroderma

A syndrome characterized by calcinosis, Raynaud's phenomenon, abnormal esophageal motility, sclerodactyly, and telangectasia (CREST) is a subset of scleroderma. Calcium deposited under the skin at the fingers or other areas oozes through the skin and releases a chalky white material. Raynaud's phenomenon is sensitivity to cold and precipitates color changes of the fingers and hands. The blood vessels go into spasm. This phenomenon was first described in 1862 by Maurice Raynaud. The hands, fingers, or just a few fingers of each hand turn white, blue, and then red. When the hands warm up, the circulation improves and the skin color returns. Raynaud's phenomenon may or may not be painful. Raynaud's phenomenon represents the first clinical sign of an altered vascular tone, and in connective tissue disease may precede other clinical symptoms by several years.

Nicotine, smoking, and cold temperatures, including those encountered in winter weather, refrigerators, and air-conditioned buildings, aggravate the condition. Smoking must be avoided. Some antihypertensive medications like nifedipine (Norvasc) dilate blood vessels and decrease the severity of the spasm. Other skin changes of scleroderma include hardening and thickening of the skin, especially the hands and fingers, arms, or face. Skin creases disappear and the skin looks shiny and tight. When this occurs over the fingers, it is difficult to make a fist or bend the fingers. Severe scleroderma results in ulcerations of the fingertips. The fingers actually shorten because of the resorption of the distal tuft of bone of the finger. The skin becomes darkened. Telangectasia of the fingers, palms, face, and lips appear as dilated tiny blood vessels near the surface of the skin. If cosmetically displeasing, dermatologists successfully treat telangectasias with laser therapy.

Swollen joints are not as common as is puffiness of the hands and feet. Arthritis and weakness are part of this disease. Fatigue will often follow. When the skin and tissues around a joint become tight, joint motion is lost and flexion contractures occur. Leathery rubs are heard as tendons move over the joints.

Early scleroderma mimics RA. Involvement of the salivary or lacrimal glands decreases secretions of the eyes and mouth. It is difficult to make tears or saliva. Dry mouth increases dental cavities. The irritation of dry eyes is a nuisance. Meticulous dental and eye care are important as preventive measures.

Gastroesophageal Reflux

The entire gastrointestinal tract is involved in scleroderma. If the lower esophageal muscles are affected, swallowing difficulties and acid reflux (GERD) occurs. Reflux causes symptoms of indigestion or heartburn. The constant reflux of acid into the esophagus creates esophagitis and esophageal stricture. Swallowing is difficult and results in vomiting or weight loss. Elevating the head of the bed, staying upright immediately after meals, and eating small portions are helpful preventive measures to avoid reflux. Proton pump inhibitors like omeprazole (Prilosec) prevent acid formation and antacids (Mylanta) minimize chronic inflammation of the esophagus. If a stricture does occur, endoscopic dilation is effective. Weakness of the walls of the colon creates large-mouthed diverticula and results in bloating, diarrhea, constipation, nausea, vomiting, and even weight loss.

Hypertension

Collagen deposition in the vessels of the kidney precipitates hypertension. Hypertension is an important prognostic indicator that results in significant complications and shortens lifespan. Hypertension must be treated quickly and aggressively.

Lung Involvement

Lung involvement occurs in more than 70 percent of patients with scleroderma and is a significant determinant of the patient's well-being. Of the patients with pulmonary fibrosis, many develop symptoms within the first few years of the illness. The deposition of collagen in the lungs interferes with the normal exchange of oxygen and carbon diox-

ide. Chest x-rays, complete pulmonary functions testing, echocardiograms, and high-resolution CT scans of the chest define lung involvement. Other testing includes heart catheterization and lavage of the lungs. There is little evidence that the fibrosis can be reversed, but corticosteroids and immunosuppression are still utilized.

As the lungs stiffen, it becomes difficult for the right ventricle to push blood through the diseased lungs. Pressures in the pulmonary artery elevate (pulmonary hypertension) and symptoms of shortness of breath develop. Eventually, heart failure occurs. Functional disability is significant and lifestyle hampered after cardiopulmonary involvement develops. Increasing shortness of breath, persistent cough, or chest pain necessitates evaluation and the need for supplemental oxygen. Lung complications are an important cause of death.

There is no treatment that will prevent collagen deposition. Instead, treatment includes the management of symptoms or complications. Infection rates increase. Newer drug therapies treat pulmonary hypertension and include epoprostenol (Flolan), bosentan (Tracleer), and prostacyclin iloprost (Ventavis Inhalant Solution). Epoprostenol relaxes blood vessels and increases the supply of blood to the lungs. This reduces the workload of the heart. Epoprostenol is administered by a continuous intravenous infusion. Bosentan is an oral tablet taken twice a day. Oral medication is more convenient, but still very expensive.

Laboratory Testing

The diagnosis of scleroderma is confirmed during a physical examination. Antibody tests are helpful. The autoantibody Scl-70 is specific to the systemic form of the disease. Routine laboratory tests evaluate vital organ functions. The biopsy of the skin is characteristic, but not often diagnostic. Other tests determine the degree of involvement of the lungs, heart, esophagus, or intestines, but are not pathognomonic. Looking at the capillaries of the nailfolds is useful to some experts. A barium swallow detects abnormalities of esophageal motility.

Treatment of Scleroderma

Early studies suggested that scleroderma improves with the antibiotic tetracycline (Minocycline). The mechanism by which this occurs is unknown and remains to be proven. Tetracycline is not universally recommended at this time until more definitive studies are completed. D-penicillamine (Depen, Cuprimine) theoretically breaks disulfide bonds between collagen and should help scleroderma patients. This has not been scientifically proven to make a blanket recommendation that all scleroderma patients receive d-penicillamine. Corticosteroids are cautiously avoided in scleroderma, although on occasion, their use becomes necessary. Other immunosuppressive agents have been utilized, including MTX or cyclophosphamide. The benefits of anti-TNF medications are being evaluated. The treatment for scleroderma is currently disappointing.

Although the cause of scleroderma remains unknown and effective therapies are lacking, the research into the understanding of the fibrosis of scleroderma has progressed. Studies show parallels with other fibrotic diseases like pulmonary fibrosis, hepatitis C, alcoholic cirrhosis, diabetes, surgical adhesions, and the restenosis of arteries following coronary angioplasty. Fibrotic diseases are all characterized by overexuberant healing by the body.

CHAPTER NINE

Bursitis/Tendinitis

A bursa is a small fluid-filled sac adjacent to the tendons and muscles. The fluid provides a cushion over prominences of bone and protects the muscles and tendons from coming into direct contact. Synovial cells line the inside surface of the bursa and the tendon sheaths. Synovial cells play a role in the inflammatory response. Bursitis and tendinitis occur as a consequence of irritation. When a bursa or tendon becomes inflamed, the synovial cells react and there is pain and swelling in the localized area. There are more than 150 bursae in the body, but the most commonly affected are the shoulders, elbows, hips, knees, and feet. Since bursitis and tendinitis mimic the same inflammatory symptoms as arthritis, they are easily confused.

The inflammation of bursitis or tendinitis is limited to the surrounding tissues about the joint, rather than the joint itself. Bursitis or tendinitis is not a chronic condition and most cases are self-limiting. Bursitis or tendinitis resolves over a short period of time, although reoccurrences are common. The inflammation starts suddenly, lasts a few days or weeks, and subsides without any permanent damage. Bursitis or tendinitis is caused by excessive pressure or incidental injury, but in most cases results from overuse or repetitive microtrauma. Repetitive microtrauma occurs while doing the same activity over and over, sometimes hundreds of times an hour or day. Bursitis and tendinitis results because of a strain, overuse in athletic events, ill-fitting shoes, or excessive activities in people already deconditioned. Older people with arthritis are more prone to bursitis than younger, conditioned individuals. Improper body mechanics irritate the bursa. Occasionally a bursa is infected.

The primary symptom of bursitis or tendinitis is pain in the affected area. The pain is dull, persistent and increases with movement. It is disturbing at night and localized. When the bursa is swollen and hot, the inflammation easily resembles infection or gout. X-rays rarely provide useful information, unless an occasional tendon calcifies. The physical exam will confirm the diagnosis. Fluid is drained from the localized area for examination and helps determine if there is infection, urate crystals, blood, or benign fluid.

Treatment and Prevention of Bursitis/Tendinitis

Mild bursitis or tendinitis is initially treated at home with rest, icing, and anti-inflammatories. If the pain is severe, disabling, or doesn't subside spontaneously, aspiration of the fluid for examination is necessary. Injection of corticosteroids relieves pain quickly. Prescription doses of NSAIDs provide relief. Surgery is rarely necessary for a troublesome bursa or tendon. Maintaining a full range of motion of the closest joint is important until the pain and inflammation resolves.

To prevent bursitis or tendonitis, activities that require repetitive motions should be avoided. Modifying activities is helpful. Conditioning makes a significant difference. If pain occurs, a particular activity should be discontinued. Intermittent rest periods, changing grips on sport racquets, avoiding prolonged overhead activities, leaning on elbows, using kneepads and safe lifting techniques, weight loss, good posture, regular exercise, and properly fitting shoes are all beneficial. Awareness of bursitis and performing regular range of motion exercises prevents many of the complications.

Hip Bursitis

Bursitis of the hip is common. Hip bursitis is uncomfortable. Pain occurs when lying in bed and rolling from side to side, putting pressure on the bursa. Tenderness to palpation occurs just over the bony prominence of the hip. Anti-inflammatories or a local steroid injection provides pain relief. X-rays rarely show any changes from normal.

Elbow Tendinitis/Bursitis

Tendinitis occurs at the muscle attachment to the outside or inside of the elbow joint (tennis or golfer's elbow). Tendinitis after tennis and other sports, gardening, or carrying heavy objects is common. Bursitis results in swelling at the elbow and can occur in conjunction with rheumatoid arthritis, gout, infection, or trauma. Bursitis at the elbow can swell significantly and resemble a golf ball.

Shoulder Tendinitis/Bursitis

Tears or inflammation of the muscles of the rotator cuff occur frequently. The rotator cuff is a group of muscles surrounding the shoulder joint. Severe pain, aching, or pain with lifting the shoulder overhead is the first sign. Rotator cuff tears are easily visualized on an MRI. A local steroid injection or anti-inflammatories help transiently. Tears of the rotator cuff are degenerative and do not heal on their own. If simple measures do not provide relief, surgical repair is necessary.

Subacromial bursitis occurs close to the same area and produces similar symptoms. Bicipital tendinitis causes pain anterior to the shoulder. The pain prevents a full range of motion. A frozen shoulder (adhesive capsulitis) occurs if the shoulder is held motionless for too long because of pain. Significant amounts of motion are lost. Adhesive capsulitis occurs quickly, but takes weeks to resolve or return to normal. Restricted motion of the shoulder makes it difficult to comb or brush the back of the head, put on coats or shirts, or put the hand in the back pocket of trousers. Range of motion exercises (pendulum exercises) must be initiated early. Occasionally patients require a general anesthetic and surgical manipulation of the shoulder to force motion and break up the adhesions about the shoulder that cause the restriction. Surgical manipulation is associated with fractures and is done only rarely, when other therapies fail.

Knee Bursitis

The anserine bursa is located just below the knee and on the inside of the leg. Pain in this area is easily confused with joint pain from the knee, although bursitis is usually well localized. Prepatellar bursitis occurs just inferior to the patella. Prepatellar bursitis is precipi-tated or aggravated by kneeling on the knee.

Foot Tendinitis

Achilles tendinitis occurs at the attachment of the Achilles tendon to the heel (calcaneous). This is a large tendon and becomes inflamed in some arthritis patients or as a result of an injury. The tendon can rupture, making it impossible to push off with the toes of the foot. Surgery is required for ruptured tendons.

Plantar fasciitis causes heel pain. The pain occurs after inactivity or upon rising in the morning. The first several steps in the morning are very tender. The heel pain of plantar fasciitis can become severely disabling. Orthotics provide extra arch support, stretching relieves tightening, and weight loss unloads extra strains from the area. Local steroid injections, oral NSAIDs, or icing are beneficial. With time, plantar fasciitis will most often subside and surgery is rarely needed.

Hand and Wrist Tendinitis

Thickening or nodule formation on the flexor tendons of the fingers results in pain, triggering, or locking. The nodule catches on the sheath that surrounds the tendon. Any finger can be involved. When a painful snap with motion occurs, the finger triggers. Rubbing the area is tender. Changing activities that cause repetitive trauma helps. Local steroid injections are useful.

Depuytren's contracture is a thickening and shortening of the fourth flexor tendon of the palm and causes one or more fingers, especially the fourth, to draw up towards the palm. It is often bilateral. Surgery is sometimes required.

DeQuervain's tenosynovitis is a painful tendinitis from overuse or inflammation of the extensor tendons of the thumb and results in pain just above the wrist. This will prevent use of the hand during simple activities like lifting a cup. Many people experiencing DeQuervain's tenosynovitis seek surgery for relief.

CHAPTER TEN

Osteoarthritis

Osteoarthritis (OA) is often called degenerative joint disease (DJD) or wear and tear arthritis. Cartilage acts as a cushion or shock absorber that pads a joint between two moving bones. Cartilage provides a smooth surface allowing movement of one bone over the other adjacent bone. OA occurs when the cartilage weakens or breaks down, leading to irregular, rough bone surfaces and deformity. Defects of the cartilage are without symptoms.

The incidence of OA increases progressively with age. Injuries, obesity, or overuse in sports or work activities puts certain joints at higher risk for developing OA. Weight-bearing joints are most often affected. OA is the most prevalent form of arthritis in the country. More than sixteen million Americans have OA. It is estimated that about sixty million Americans will have OA by the year 2020. About equal numbers of men and women have OA. The onset and symptoms occur most commonly after the age of forty-five. OA is a major source of disability in the elderly, potentially equaling that associated with cardiovascular disease or stroke. OA disables as much as 6 percent of the general population. Five percent of those over the age of fifty-five will experience OA of the hip, and half of these patients will ultimately require hip replacement. Most individuals over sixty have evidence of OA on x-ray.

Clinical Symptoms of OA

Patients experience pain localized to the joint without the signs of inflammation seen in other joint diseases like RA. The pain is worse with activity and relieved by rest. As the disease progresses, pain occurs with very little motion, even at rest. The pain is described as deep, aching, and poorly localized. Pain comes on slowly as the joint space changes and pain fibers around the joint are irritated.

Any joint may be involved, but the most frequently affected are the weight-bearing joints like the hips, knees, and spine. Involvement of the knee is likely to result in significant disability. X-rays changes are characteristic as compared to other inflammatory types of arthritis and reveal irregular narrowing of the joint space, spurs (osteophytes), sclerosis, and subchondral cysts. OA is characterized by bony growth. Laboratory studies in OA are normal, including measurements of inflammation like the erythrocyte sedimentation rate (ESR) or C-reactive protein (CRP).

Typical X-ray Changes of Osteoarthritis
◊ sclerosis
◊ irregular narrowing of the joint
◊ osteophytes
◊ subchondral cysts

Hands

No one knows why one person gets OA and another doesn't. Heredity plays an important role. Heberden's nodes are the bony enlargements of the distal interphalangeal joint (DIP). The nodes are firm, hard, bony enlargements occurring slowly over time. On occasion Heberden's nodes come on more rapidly and are inflammatory. They may contain gelatinous material and form cysts. When inflamed, they are painful. Later, the nodes enlarge and are usually not painful. The joint is stiff, but function is not impaired. Rarely do the DIPs require surgery.

Heberden's nodes are more common in women and are more likely to occur in female relatives. Nodal formation of the proximal interphalangeal joint (PIP) is a Bouchard node and is also characteristic of OA. OA at the base of the thumb of the first carpal metacarpal joint results in a squared off appearance and is very symptomatic. Local corticosteroid injections provide transient relief. NSAIDs help and surgery on occasion is required.

Lower Extremities

Stiffness after periods of immobility characterizes OA of the knee or hip. The stiffness usually lasts less than thirty minutes, compared to the stiffness of RA, which may last all day. Joint stiffness is exacerbated by weather changes. In OA, the joint fluid gels and contributes to the stiffness.

The pain of the hip is localized early to the groin or referred to the knee. Hip pain may be confused with knee pain and difficult to differentiate. Limping is common. Crossing the legs is difficult. Severe OA of the hip makes personal hygiene difficult. Getting off the commode can be impossible. In elderly individuals, hip replacement is needed to help with ambulation, but also to ease with transfers, self-care, and hygiene.

OA of the knee is aggravated by activities that require increased motion, especially squatting, climbing, or walking. Walking downstairs is more difficult than going up. Weight bearing is painful. Crepitation is often detectable. Swelling of the knee is common, and fluid can fill the entire joint space. Increased pressure in the front of the knee sends the fluid to the back of the knee, forming a popliteal cyst (Baker's cyst). The joint gets tight, making it difficult to fully extending the knee. The fluid no longer goes back to the front of the knee because of a ball and valve mechanism that creates a one-way valve effect. The cyst gets bigger, tighter, and ruptures. Fluid abruptly travels down the leg, mimicking deep-vein phlebitis (DVT). A ruptured popliteal cyst is painful and creates swelling of the calf and leg. Ruptured popliteal cysts are more common in inflammatory forms of arthritis than OA because more fluid accumulates within the joint.

Any swelling or pain of the knee results in atrophy of the quadriceps muscles above the knee within a few days. When muscles are weak, the knee is at an increased risk for injury. Months of regular exercise are necessary to gain back the muscle strength lost in just a few days. Immobility and persistent flexion encourages a fixed flexion deformity of the knee. Knee flexion contractures make ambulation difficult, require more

muscle strength, and put tremendous energy demands on the individual.

OA Variants

Variants of OA exist. Primary inflammatory OA of the small joints of the fingers resembles RA. Diffuse idiopathic skeletal hyperostosis (DISH) involves the anterior portion of the spine with flowing calcification of the anterior longitudinal ligament. When DISH occurs in the cervical area, the calcification can be large enough to interfere with swallowing. OA is associated with calcium pyrophosphate deposition disease (CPPD) or pseudogout. Pseudogout is acute or chronic and typically involves knees, wrists, and shoulders. The crystal of CPPD precipitates inflammation. The response to treatment and the natural course of pseudogout is distinctly different from gout. In the elderly, pseudogout is to the knee as gout is to the big toe.

Treatment of OA

There is no known cause or cure for OA. The treatment is both nonpharmacologic and pharmacologic. Patient education is an integral part of the treatment program. Treatment is tailored to an individual's needs to reduce pain, maintain and/or improve joint mobility, and limit functional disability. Proper use of a cane on the opposite side of a diseased hip or knee teaches the patient to reduce the loading forces on the joint and is associated with decreased pain and improved function. The cane should be of a proper height and length. When the person is standing erect, with arms to the sides, the top of a curved handled cane or the level part if a straight handled cane should come to the level of the wrist crease.

Acetaminophen (Tylenol) should be the first drug used in the treatment of OA. Later, NSAIDs and mild non-narcotic analgesics form the basis of drug therapy. No drug therapy is known to change the course of the disease or slow its progress. Oral steroids are rarely used. Occasional intra-articular steroids provide rapid and significant relief. Corticosteroid injections are justifiable for temporary and immediate relief, but should be done judiciously. Viscosupplementation is a series of intra-articular injections of hyluronan or hyaluronic acid into the knee joint space. Hyaluronic acid is a natural constituent of joint fluid that provides a natural cushioning effect within the joint. Without hyaluronic acid, the fluid loses its elastic and viscosity properties. If the degenerative changes of the knee are not too severe, a series of hyaluronic injections into the knee joint space provide six to twelve months of pain relief. Viscosupplementation has been done with success into other joints, but currently remains unapproved by the FDA.

Current hyaluronic agents include Orthovisc, Synvisc, Supartz, Euflexxa, and Hyalgan. There are some important differences among these agents. Since deterioration of the cartilage is central to OA, current research is looking at the biochemical metabolism of cartilage. With very little scientific proof, a number of unproven remedies have been suggested to improve the metabolism of cartilage. At this time, these remedies cannot be uniformly recommended.

Prognosis of OA

The prognosis is good for OA. The disease progresses slowly and stabilizes without significant changes for years. Good lifestyle habits make a difference in the final outcome. Exercise helps maintain muscle strength, body weight, and general health. Swimming is best for those individuals with involvement of weight-bearing joints, but walking, and even resistance exercise, helps build muscle strength and improve range of motion. When conservative therapy fails, surgical intervention is of significant benefit.

CHAPTER ELEVEN

Muscle

Muscle inflammation (myositis) results in weakness. Polymyositis (PM) and dermatomyositis (DM) are myopathies closely related to other autoimmune diseases.

Polymyositis

Polymyositis is a disease characterized by inflammation of most muscles. The weakness occurs in proximal muscles (closer to the trunk) more than distal muscles (away from the trunk), especially shoulders, upper arms, thighs, and hips, in a symmetrical pattern. The peak onset is between the ages of thirty and sixty years, but PM can affect children and people over sixty. Involvement of the neck or chest muscles makes it difficult to breath, swallow, or lift the head. Systemic symptoms include fever, weight loss, general malaise, muscle pain (myalgia) and less commonly joint pain (arthralgias). Muscle weakness can be profound or subtle. Like other collagen vascular disease, patients with PM have a detectable ANA.

Prompt treatment includes anti-inflammatories, corticosteroids, intravenous immunoglobulin (IVIG), and immunosuppressants. Therapy can reverse or at least prevent progression of muscle weakness. Corticosteroid-related problems occur frequently during treatment and contribute significantly to the functional disability reported by myositis patients. Significant doses of corticosteroids contribute to corticosteroid myopathy and weakness that confuses response to therapy. Corticosteroid myopathy requires the immediate lowering of the corticosteroid dose.

Dermatomyositis

Dermatomyositis is similar to PM. The muscle inflammation of DM is accompanied by skin inflammation. Dermatomyositis combines an inflammatory myopathy associated with a characteristic skin rash. DM is closely related to PM and is a spectrum of the same disease. Both PM and DM are collagen vascular diseases and coincide with other connective tissue diseases like lupus.

Dermatomyositis may be associated with malignancy. The association of malignancy with PM is perhaps coincidental. Cancer is considered in those individuals with DM who fail to respond to therapy. Removing or treating the cancer eliminates the effect on the muscles. A heliotrope rash is a dark symmetrical violaceous discoloration around the eyes occurring in DM. The rash is obvious or subtle and associated with swelling around the eyes. Bumps over bony prominences of the knuckles of the hands or knees are elevated and violaceous (Gottron's Sign). Initial complaints include weakness and fatigue. Climbing stairs is difficult or impossible. The inability to swallow suggests more serious involvement. Progression of the disease is slow or rapid over days or months.

Laboratory abnormalities are typical of PM or DM. Muscle enzyme elevations of creatinine phosphokinase (CPK) or aldolase are easy to measure. Abnormal electrical conductivity of the muscles is measured by electromyography (EMG). Distinctive muscle biopsies characterize both diseases, but require detailed and expert examination of the muscle, occasionally by electron microscopy. The muscle enzyme elevations are dramatic and are used to monitor disease activity and response to therapy.

Criteria for the Diagnosis of Muscle Inflammation
◊ proximal and symmetrical muscle weakness
◊ lab evidence of muscle inflammation
◊ muscle enzyme elevation
◊ abnormal electromyogram
◊ abnormal muscle biopsy
◊ abnormal magnetic resonance imaging
◊ characteristic skin changes

Inclusion-Body Myositis

Inclusion-body myositis is characterized by a unique biopsy best seen on electron microscopy. Inclusion-body myositis (IBM) patients have proximal and symmetric weakness that does not respond well to therapy. Inclusion-body myositis occurs in men more than women. Signs of IBM usually start after age fifty. A small number of IBM cases may be hereditary. Inclusion-body myositis develops slower than other types of myositis. Muscle weakness happens over months or years.

Drugs and Myopathy

Many lipid-lowering agents (statins) cause muscle weakness, elevated muscle enzymes, and myalgia. The exact mechanism and cause is still not well understood. Severe inflammation and destruction of the muscle is unusual. Withdrawal of the drug results in relief of muscle pain, return of strength, and return to normal CPK levels. Persistent symptoms or elevations of CPK may unmask a different myopathy and require further testing or treatment. Laboratory tests and a muscle biopsy with special staining are required. An experienced surgeon is required to do the biopsy. The specimen must be handled carefully and sent to a center for electron microscopy. Muscle biopsies are done after the EMG. The EMG will locate the best muscle site to biopsy. Doing the EMG on one side of the body and a muscle biopsy on the other side avoids artifact created by the EMG needles.

Thyroid disease, enzyme and metabolic deficiencies of muscles, and inherited illnesses can mimic inflammatory muscle disease. The EMG, elevated muscle enzymes, and strength all gauge response to treatment.

Treatment of Myositis

Regardless of the cause, general measures are important in treating patients with myopathy. Bed rest is valuable. Rest is combined with range of motion exercises to prevent contractures of the joints and preserve function. The mainstay of treatment includes corticosteroids and/or intravenous immunoglobulin (IVIG). Antimalarial drugs are useful in a few patients. The overall prognosis varies, but intervention makes a difference and full recoveries are possible. Almost all patients will respond to high doses of steroids. As elevated muscle enzyme levels return to normal, the weakness abates. Normal strength will return. Immunosuppressive agents like methotrexate or azathioprine are useful in those individuals with disease refractory to corticosteroids or in those patients experiencing unacceptable side effects of corticosteroids. Immunosuppressive agents help lower the dose of corticosteroids.

CHAPTER TWELVE

Vasculitis

Vasculitis   is an inflammation of the arterial blood vessels. Small, medium, or large arteries are affected. Inflammation results in leakage of blood from the vessel, tender nodularity, and obstruction of the normal blood flow. If blood flow is obstructed, the tissue dies and gangrene occurs. In connective tissue diseases, immune complexes deposit in the blood vessel wall. Immune complexes create inflammation and swelling, harm the vessel wall, and interfere with normal blood flow. In small vessels, vasculitis quickly becomes important and painful. Fingertips become gangrenous. Surgery, or even amputation, becomes necessary for severely compromised areas.

Clinical Findings of Vasculitis

Depending on the blood vessels involved, vasculitis causes many different symptoms and findings. Systemic symptoms include fever, malaise, poor appetite, weight loss, and fatigue. Small petechiae appear on the legs. Large areas of purpura resemble bruising. Nailfold infarcts occur on the tip of the finger or around the fingernails. Pitting scars of the fingertips result as a consequence of infarcts. Other symptoms include joint pains, headache, behavioral disturbance, confusion, seizures, and stroke. Neuropathy as a consequence of vasculitis causes symptoms of pain, sensitivity, numbness, tingling, diminished sensation, or loss of strength. Heart attacks result as a consequence of coronary vasculitis. Lung involvement resembles pneumonia. Other areas of involvement include the eyes, kidneys, and intestines.

Hypersensitivity vasculitis is associated with drug reactions or other connective tissue disease. Systemic necrotizing vasculitis affects many organ systems and is life threatening. Other forms of vasculitis include polyarteritis nodosa, Churge-Strauss syndrome, or Wegener's granulomatosis. Signs or symptoms are highly variable and the diagnosis is challenging. A biopsy of tissue is often required and diagnostic. Immune mechanisms result in characteristic laboratory findings.

Treatment of Vasculitis

The goal of the treatment of vasculitis is the suppression of the inflammatory response (immunosuppression). Treatment includes corticosteroids, cytotoxic drugs such as cyclophosphamide (Cytoxan), or plasmapheresis. Plasmapheresis is an alternative method to remove circulating immune complexes from the circulation. During plasmapheresis, whole blood is removed and spun in an apparatus that separates the different cellular components from the plasma. Since the plasma contains the immune complexes that stimulate the inflammatory response, the plasma is discarded. Cytotoxic drugs are given concurrently. Treatment regimes play an important role in the final outcome of the disease and are continued for prolonged periods.

Cyclophosphamide is the drug of choice for the treatment of vasculitis. Daily oral dosing results in bone marrow suppression and low blood counts. The dose is adjusted based on the results of frequent blood counts. Oversuppression of the bone marrow is significant and puts patients at risk for infection. All cytotoxic drugs can precipitate serious adverse effects. Doses are kept to a minimum to induce remission and obtain the desired effects. Cyclophosphamide is associated with an increased incidence in cancer and hemorrhagic bleeding of the bladder. Encouraging fluid intake and diluting the effects of cyclophosphamide in the urine avoids hemorrhagic cystitis.

Azathioprine (Imuran) is another immunosuppressive agent and has some advantages. Azathioprine is not associated with gonadal suppression, sterility, or significant potential to induce cancer. Blood counts are suppressed by azathioprine, and there is still an increased risk for infection.

Mycophenolate (Cellcept) was originally used in the management of patients with organ transplants. Today mycophenolate is often used in the treatment of autoimmune disorders, and it is useful to treat lupus nephritis. Mycophenolate targets an enzyme step that is critical to the formation of DNA. By interfering with DNA, the medication impairs overactive immune cells of lupus. In adults, mycophenolate is given twice daily (2000 to 3000 milligrams/daily), given with food to help to prevent nausea or stomach pain. Mycophenolate is supplied as 250-milligram and 500-milligram capsules or tablets. Regular blood tests are necessary.

The effects of immunosuppressive drug therapy during pregnancy are not well studied. Young women must use effective birth control while taking these medications.

Giant Cell Arteritis

Giant cell arteritis (GCA) is an inflammatory condition of large- and medium-sized arteries affecting the branches of the carotid arteries. It is also called temporal arteritis because of the involvement of the temporal artery. The temporal artery is easily palpated. Since GCA results in permanent blindness, early treatment is a medical emergency. Patients develop permanent blindness because of inflammation of the optic artery. Giant cell arteritis typically occurs in people over the age of fifty and is more common in women than in men.

Since the same patient population develops polymyalgia rheumatica (PMR) and GCA, these conditions may be a spectrum of the same disease. Frequently, the two illnesses occur in the same individual. These two conditions are likely to have the same cause, but the reason why some people have only one syndrome and others both is still unknown. At least half of the people with GCA also have polymyalgia rheumatica. Both GCA and PMR will resolve spontaneously within two years of onset and rarely return. In GCA, symptoms include headache, especially over the temporal area of the head, jaw pain with chewing, fever, and scalp tenderness. The symptoms of GCA must be taken seriously.

Criteria for Giant Cell or Temporal Arteritis
◊ age at onset of symptoms over fifty years old
◊ new headache and localized pain in the temple
◊ temporal artery tenderness to palpitation
◊ elevated sedimentation rate greater than fifty
◊ an abnormal temporal artery biopsy

Treatment of Giant Cell Arteritis

Treatment with high-dose (>60 milligrams of prednisone daily) oral corticosteroids prevents visual disturbances, but must be started at the onset of the first symptoms. Side effects secondary to corticosteroids always occur. Occasionally, cytotoxic drug therapy and other immunosuppressives are necessary. Unfortunately, the elderly population of GCA is already dealing with problems of osteoporosis, cataracts, hypertension, or other problems that high-dose corticosteroids aggravate. It is important to be sure that the treatment is not worse than the disease. Corticosteroids are required for extended periods of time and are monitored by the ESR. Patients take concurrent calcium supplements, multivitamins, and bisphosphonates to protect against steroid-induced osteoporosis. A bone density measurement is done at the initiation of prolonged corticosteroid therapy.

Polymyalgia Rheumatica

Polymyalgia Rheumatica (PMR) is characterized by aching and morning stiffness in the upper portions of the muscles and joints of the arms and legs in a symmetrical fashion. It is common and occurs in individuals over fifty years of age. The symptoms are often vague and difficult to describe. Fatigue and weight loss occur commonly. Symptoms of PMR occur in the shoulder and pelvic girdles. There is almost always evidence of an elevated ESR. The onset may be abrupt, but in most instances the symptoms are present for weeks or months and elude a definitive early diagnosis.

Criteria for Polymyalgia Rheumatica
◊ elderly
◊ aching and morning stiffness
◊ shoulder girdle involvement
◊ pelvic girdle involvement
◊ elevated sedimentation rate
◊ mild anemia

Comparing GCA and PMR

There is evidence of mild anemia and mild abnormalities on the chemistry panel in both GCA and PMR. The only significant laboratory abnormality in both is a markedly elevated ESR. The ESR changes with the activity of the disease and response to treatment. The ESR relates to disease activity better than the patient or physician's impression. It is measured frequently during the course of the disease. A normal ESR is less than twenty, but extremely elevated ESRs are not uncommon and can be over one hundred at the time of diagnosis.

The diagnosis of GCA is confirmed by a biopsy of the temporal artery. Temporal artery biopsy is a relatively safe and easy procedure done in an outpatient setting. Most often, only one artery is biopsied. Biopsies are not repeated to monitor response to treatment; instead, clinical symptoms and the ESR are followed. In GCA, the microscopic biopsy findings are segmental and require a thorough examination of a long segment of artery. The demonstration of giant cells confirms the diagnosis. In PMR, the arteries are not involved and not biopsied. X-rays show no specific findings.

Giant cell arteritis requires that treatment be initiated with a high dose of prednisone (60 milligrams equivalent/daily) and then tapered slowly over months, depending on symptoms and the ESR. The primary reason for a high dose of corticosteroid is to prevent blindness. Unfortunately, the GCA population is elderly, and the side effects secondary to corticosteroids are significant.

Polymyalgia rheumatica is treated

with lower doses of prednisone (20 milligrams/daily) and tapered slowly over two years. A dramatic response to low-dose corticosteroid therapy within twenty-four hours is characteristic of PMR. The day after the first oral dose of steroid, a physician or a nurse doesn't need to ask how the patient feels. Patients offer a spontaneous and immediate positive response. The results are so striking that patients immediately resume their usual activities. Polymyalgia rheumatica often mimics RA, especially in those individuals with a negative rheumatoid factor. Both GCA and PMR run a self-limited course and will resolve. Patients treated for less than two years with prednisone have a high relapse rate. A small proportion of patients need steroids for an extended period of time.

It is recognized that the complications of the corticosteroids are substantial in the elderly. Osteoporosis is one of the side effects of most concern. A baseline bone density measurement is done and calcium and vitamin D supplements started at the same time corticosteroids are initiated. If corticosteroids are continued for a prolonged period of time, bisphosphonates are started to prevent osteoporosis. Alternate-day corticosteroids are usually not as effective as daily oral doses. Catastrophic complications of the disease are infrequent with treatment. The ESR and clinical symptoms are monitored while corticosteroids are tapered slowly. During relapses in either disease, the ESR increases with the recurrence of symptoms. The ESR is the best test to monitor the disease. Both illnesses rarely occur when a normal ESR is measured.

CHAPTER THIRTEEN

Sjogren's Syndrome

Sjogren's syndrome (SS) is an autoimmune disorder associated with dry eyes and mouth (keratoconjunctivitis sicca). Primary SS occurs by itself and is not associated with other diseases. Secondary SS occurs with other rheumatic diseases. Most patients are women, although SS affects adults of any age or ethnic background. The Arthritis Foundation estimates that more than one million people in the United States have SS.

Although SS is a systemic illness like other rheumatic illnesses, SS is characterized more by the loss of tears in the eyes and saliva in the mouth than other rheumatic illnesses. Vaginal dryness also occurs. Lymphocytes invade the glands of the eyes and mouth. The glands become nonfunctional and eventually do not produce tears or secretions.

Dryness Symptoms of Sjogren's Syndrome
◊ dry mouth
◊ nasal dryness
◊ vaginal dryness
◊ dry skin

The lymphocytes infiltrate the salivary glands, cause pain and swelling, and mimic lymphoma. On occasion a biopsy is necessary to differentiate SS from more serious disease. Lymphoma occurs more frequently in individuals with SS than in those without SS. Since treatment is often conservative, invasive or more sophisticated testing is not always necessary. A lip biopsy is diagnostic, but uncomfortable. Biopsies are seldom done. More sophisticated tests can be done to determine salivary gland function or tear production. Specialized blood markers detect antibodies that are specific for SS, especially the Sjogren's syndrome autoantibody (SSA). Not every patient will have detectable antibodies. Opthalmalogical examination looks carefully for either the absence of tears or the harm done as a consequence of dry eyes. Routine examinations determine systemic involvement and other connective disease like RA.

Treatment of Sjogren's Syndrome

The cause of SS is not known. There is no cure or specific therapy. Fortunately, SS is not usually a life-threatening illness. The treatment of the associated rheumatic illness should occur first. Eye infections are treated promptly. Sipping water throughout the day is helpful for dry mouth. Sucking on sugar-free hard candies provides some relief and stimulates saliva production. Meticulous dental care is crucial and follow-up with dental professionals for regular dental hygiene is important. Treatment is designed to relieve discomfort and prevent any damage from the effects of dryness.

Artificial tears relieve the dry scratchy discomfort of the eyes during the day. Other products like lubricants or longer-acting inserts are available. On occasion the ophthalmologist can block the canal of the eye that drains tears. This helps retain tears and moisturizes the eyes longer. Vaginal lubricants help vaginal dryness and lessen discomfort. Pilocarpine (Salagen) tablets (5 milligrams four times daily) stimulate the salivary glands and production of saliva. Cevimeline (Evoxac) is similar. The effect of Evoxac at 30 milligrams lasts only three to five hours. In clinical trials, efficacy was established at six weeks with cevimeline. The most common side effect of either drug is sweating. Other symptoms include chills, flushing, and frequent urination. Artificial saliva products include Glandosane (non-aerosol spray), Moist Stir Oral Swab Sticks (pretreated swabs), MouthKote (non-aerosol spray), Oralube (liquid to swish in mouth), Salivert (aerosol spray), and Xero-Lube Artificial Saliva (non-aerosol spray). Cyclosporine ophthalmic drops (Restasis) will increase the tear production of those individuals who have suppressed tear production secondary to keratoconjunctivitis sicca.

CHAPTER FOURTEEN

Joint Infections

Individuals with chronic forms of arthritis are at an increased risk for bacterial infection within the joint. Acute infection must be considered when the inflammation of a single joint in a patient with chronic arthritis is out of proportion to the other joints. Most septic joints are bacterial in origin. Immunosuppressed individuals are at risk for opportunistic and unusual infections like tuberculosis or fungal infections.

Reactive arthritis occurs as a response to an infection elsewhere in the body. Joint symptoms are inflammatory and characterized by extreme pain, erythema, swelling, and warmth. Gram stains contain no organisms and cultures are sterile. Several infections that never reside within the joint space manifest themselves primarily as arthritis. The bacteria most often associated with reactive arthritis are chlamydia (*Chlamydia trachomatis*) and are usually acquired through sexual contact. Infections in the digestive tract that may trigger reactive arthritis include the bacteria *Salmonella, Shigella, Yersinia,* and *Campylobacter.* Infections occur after eating or handling improperly prepared food. Most patients with reactive arthritis test positive for the genetic marker HLA-B27.

Bacterial Infections

Bacterial joint infections occur as a result of the hematogenous spread (blood) of bacteria entering the joint. Septic joints are more common in joints already affected by arthritis. Infections of joints in young, healthy individuals are much less common. Bacteria most often enter through the upper respiratory tract, gastrointestinal tract, or skin. Surgically replaced joints are at increased risk for bacterial infection. Venereal disease, tuberculosis, streptococcal infections, and other infections can all cause septic joints at distant sites far from the site of the original infection. Most bacterial joint infections require hospitalization, surgical drainage, and intravenous antibiotics. Needle aspiration of an infected joint fluid is diagnostic, but only seldom therapeutic. Arthroscopy and synovectomy may be necessary. Acute bacterial infection of the joint is usually associated with fevers and chills. The pain and swelling within the joint are severe. Individuals taking chronic corticosteroid have an increased risk for bacterial infection and a blunted response to infection. Bacterial infection of a joint is a medical emergency. Fungal infections are indolent and smolder as compared to an acute bacterial infection.

Viral Infections

Viral causes of arthritis include hepatitis, mumps, mononucleosis, or other viral illnesses like measles. The rubella vaccine has been associated with a reaction similar to arthritis. Viral causes of arthritis are often the result of the immune response to the infection. The effect of the virus creates an immune reaction within the joint. As the viral infection resolves, so does the arthritis. There is usually low-grade fever, headache, photophobia, and muscle pain (myalgia). Antibiotics are not effective treatment.

Fungal Infections

Fungal infections are uncommon in healthy individuals, but are more common in those individuals with a suppressed immune status like intravenous drug abusers, cancer patients, corticosteroid treated patients, and patients with alcoholism, anemia, chronic illness like arthritis, diabetes, or AIDS. Infectious arthritis as a result of a fungus is often resistant to treatment and requires surgical intervention and months of drug therapy. Recurrence is possible. The infection is not always as inflammatory or obvious as the infections associated with bacteria. A biopsy of synovial tissue may be required to establish the diagnosis.

Lyme Disease

Lyme disease is a bacterial infection transmitted by the bite of an infected deer tick. The bite of the deer tick carries the bacterium *Borrelia burgdorferi*. The first reported cases occurred in Old Lyme, Connecticut. Now, most areas in the United States have reported Lyme disease, but it is more common in certain areas of the country, especially the Northeast and Middle Atlantic states, California, and Oregon. The arthritis is treated with antibiotics. Most cases are reported in the spring and summer months, when ticks are the most active and people are outdoors.

Early symptoms within a week of a tick bite include a flu-like illness. Arthralgias and myalgias occur with fever, chills, fatigue, and headache. At the site of the tick bite, a characteristic rash occurs. It often looks like a "bull's eye" that includes a red ring with a clear center (erythema migrans) that expands and enlarges slowly over several days. Either the rash or actual tick bite can go unnoticed. If left untreated, Lyme disease causes more serious nerve or heart problems and can mimic other conditions, making the diagnosis difficult. For most people, symptoms will resolve on their own within a few months without treatment. Specialized laboratory testing can confirm lyme disease.

Chronic arthritis resembling RA results as a consequence of Lyme disease. Only about 10 percent of those infected will develop arthritis. In those individuals visiting or living in areas that are at risk, it is important to consider Lyme disease as a cause of arthritis otherwise unexplained, especially arthritis characterized by attacks in a few large joints like the knees.

Early antibiotic treatment is generally successful. Administration of doxycycline (100 milligrams twice daily) or amoxicillin (500 milligrams three times daily) for fourteen to twenty-one days is recommended for treatment of early localized or early-disseminated Lyme disease associated with erythema migrans. Treatment prevents more serious involvement. Laboratory tests are available to confirm the infection in those individuals that have either physical findings or a history to suggest they are at risk for Lyme disease.

The best treatment of Lyme disease is avoidance of tick bites. With active outdoor living, precautions and awareness of potential tick bites becomes important. The tick is very small and is easily missed. Small children and adults should inspect for tick bites after time spent outdoors. Using a tick repellent, protective clothing, and avoiding brush or other areas where ticks come in contact with people lessens the chance of an infection. Ticks are found in tall grasses in marshes or fields and in the brush in wooded areas. Ticks are easily picked up on clothing or skin.

Precautions to Help Avoid Lyme Disease

◊ Wear long pants while in grasses or brush.
◊ Spray before going out in potential spaces where ticks reside.
◊ Inspect yourself when coming in from tick-infested areas.

Parvovirus

Erythema infectiosum or fifth disease is the most common manifestation of parvovirus B19 infection and occurs commonly in school-age children. It presents as a mild febrile illness with a red rash of variable intensity. The early rosy to bright red "slapped cheek" appearance is often overlooked. Eventually a lacy, net-like redness develops that involves the face, arms, and trunk. In adults, the rash is less common, but the joint involvement resembles a polyarthritis like RA. Evidence of previous parvovirus B19 infection in the serum is common among adults. The laboratory studies sort out acute versus previous old infections. Most forms of this arthritis will resolve without intervention and without any permanent impairment.

Rheumatic Fever

Rheumatic fever follows a sore throat secondary to an infection with streptococcus bacteria. If the infection isn't treated early enough, rheumatic fever may follow. Symptoms in children usually include fever, arthritis, and inflammation of the heart. In some cases, this inflammation leads to rheumatic heart disease. People who experience arthritis as the dominant symptom may experience recurrent arthritis flares later in life. As yet, there is no definitive laboratory test to identify rheumatic fever, but there are laboratory studies to confirm streptococcal infections. The diagnosis is based primarily on the evaluation of clinical signs and symptoms. Evidence of a preceding infection in the laboratory is required to make the diagnosis. Although children are at most risk between the ages of seven and ten, adults also get rheumatic fever. In adults, arthritis is the most important manifestation and in children, the heart inflammation. Patients respond to high doses of aspirin for several weeks. Antibiotics are given for the streptococcal infection.

Hepatitis

There are a number of viruses responsible for inflammation of the liver, including hepatitis A, B, and C. An associated antibody response by the immune system preceding or during an episode of hepatitis is responsible for many effects on the musculoskeletal system. Arthritis or arthralgia occurs before there is clinical evidence of hepatitis or jaundice. Symptoms usually resolve by the time the patient is jaundiced. Hepatitis can result in a false positive test for rheumatoid factor.

AIDS

Arthritis has been associated with human immunodeficiency virus. Initial HIV infection is associated with a flu-like illness. Some patients experience a painful articular syndrome. Whether Reiter's syndrome, psoriatic arthritis, or other reactive arthritis is more prevalent in HIV infected individuals remains controversial.

Rubella

Like other viral infections, rubella is associated with arthralgias or arthritis. In most patients, symptoms are short-lived, but in some individuals symptoms last for years. Joint symptoms occur just before or shortly after rash develops. Vaccines for rubella contain live attenuated virus. A high frequency of post-vaccination joint pain, muscle pain, and arthritis follows the vaccination. Symptoms occur shortly after the vaccination, but then resolve spontaneously over several days.

Pneumococcal Disease

Pneumococcal disease is an infection caused by bacteria. It is not associated with arthritis, but there is an added risk in people with arthritis and an impaired immune system. Vaccination (Pneumovax) protects from this potentially life-threatening infection. There are three general types of infection. Upper respiratory infections affecting the middle ear or sinuses, lower respiratory tract infections including pneumonia, and invasive infections like sepsis or meningitis. Annually, pneumococcal infections are responsible for more deaths than any other vaccine preventable bacterial disease. One-half of these deaths could have been prevented by use of the vaccine. All patients with chronic forms of arthritis should have a pneumococcal vaccination and booster every five years.

Antibiotic Principles

The overuse of antibiotics is dangerous and accelerates the rate of development of drug-resistant bacteria. Individuals with rheumatic illnesses have an increased risk for infections, but not all necessarily require antibiotics. Viral infections do not require antibiotics. Many patients insist on taking antibiotic therapy for anything that resembles infection. For patients on immunosuppressive drug therapy, this is reasonable. Even so, it is important that basic principles be followed. Since narrow spectrum antibiotics will be less likely to force bacteria to mutate and selectively allow resistant bacteria to flourish, narrow spectrum antibiotics should always be used. Underdosing of antibiotics is avoided, since this encourages development of resistant strains of bacteria, too.

CHAPTER FIFTEEN

How Joints Are Affected

Joint Space

A microscopic membrane of synovial cells lines the joint cavity. The joint cavity is filled with a small amount of synovial fluid. The fluid is clear or slightly yellow. Synovitis is synonymous with the term arthritis. The synovial cells in inflammatory arthritis multiply and go from a few cell layers thick to hundreds of cell layers thick. Rather than blocking the movement of fluid and cells from the blood into the joint space, the synovial pannus that is formed allows fluid to come into the joint cavity. The joint swells and is painful. The fluid contains inflammatory white cells, chemical mediators of inflammation (cytokines), and enzymes (metalloproteases) that promote harmful reactions to the cartilage. Damage to the cartilage occurs and results in arthritis.

The typical joint is surrounded by a fibrous capsule that forms a joint space. Each end of the bone is covered with cartilage, which forms a smooth, glistening surface and functions as a cushion. Cartilage allows the bones to slide against each other with minimal friction. Cartilage is radiolucent and does not show on x-ray, but is visible on sophisticated studies like magnetic resonance imaging. The width of the joint space on the x-ray helps estimate the thickness of the remaining cartilage. Weight-bearing x-rays of the knee are useful to determine estimates of the size of joint space and the amount of cartilage remaining.

The movement of the joints depends on the muscles and tendons that are outside the joint space. The knee has fibrous bands or ligaments within the joint space that can be injured. Blood vessels are outside the joint space. During inflammatory arthritis or an injury, fluid from the blood easily moves into the joint space and out. Extreme swelling or a large effusion within the joint space creates intense pain.

Hip

Most forms of arthritis attack the ball (femoral head) and socket joint (acetabulum) of the hip. The hips are most often affected by OA. Other forms of inflammatory arthritis and injuries occur at the hip. Disease occurs in one hip or both. Congenital dysplasia of the hip may result in OA, but it is not recognized until later in life. The blood supply to the hip is unique and subject to injury or interruption. Avascular necrosis (AVN) of the femoral head results in necrosis of bone and disruption of the joint. Early hip pain occurs in the groin. Later, walking is painful in the entire hip region. Pain may radiate down the leg and mimic knee pain. Fortunately, total hip replacement (THR) is quite successful. Avascular necrosis may occur in other sites than the hip.

Total hip replacement is currently one of the most widely performed procedures in general orthopedic practice today. Since its introduction in 1969, it has proved remarkably successful in eliminating pain and restoring function of the hips. Newer hip replacements will likely last a lifetime. Over 70 percent of THRs are done for OA. These people have failed to find relief in conservative management for pain and experience limitation in their activities of daily living. It is generally preferred that THR be done in those individuals over sixty years of age. At this age, the physical demands on the prosthesis are less.

The longevity of the metal prosthesis approaches the life expectancy of the patient and avoids the need for revision. Regardless, this procedure is done at any age.

Indications for Total Hip Replacement
◊ pain at night
◊ severe pain limiting activities of daily living
◊ pain requiring increasing amounts of narcotics
◊ pain preventing daily fun and light activities

Knee

The knee has the distinction of being the most problematic joint. There are many reasons why the knee creates so much trouble. The knee is the largest weight-bearing joint. The knee is also the most complex joint. There are a number of internal structures within the knee that allow it to have many motions. Arthritis is the end result of injury and abuse over years.

Excessive weight adds to the abuse of the knees. It creates more problems than any other factor. Both knees support the total body weight. Exercise plays both a positive and negative role in the abuse and deterioration of the knees. A swollen knee loses strength in the quadriceps

Knee Replacement

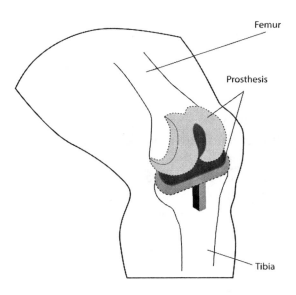

muscles within a few days of onset of swelling and is visibly smaller compared to the opposite (contralateral) side just as quickly. Exercising the quadriceps muscles protects the knee, primarily by diminishing stress and pain of the knee. The most comfortable position for any swollen joint is flexion. Flexion lessens the pain and discomfort, but encourages a fixed flexion deformity. During acute inflammation of the knee, continuous rest and flexion is discouraged. When pain is controlled, early active range of motion will preserve function.

Arthritis behind the patella (chondromalacia patella) causes inflammation and pain of the knee. As much as one third of the population has isolated ar-

thritis under the patella. It is twice as common in women as in men. Most individuals do all their activities, but at the end of the day experience pain, swelling, or stiffness as the fluid within the knee space accumulates and gels. A great deal of fluid causes throbbing nocturnal knee pain. Going downstairs, rather than going up, is aggravated by patellofemoral arthritis. In chondromalacia patella, the patella does not track through the largest space of the femur, where there is the most room.

This malalignment theory has led to surgical procedures and strategies to realign patellar tracking. Outcomes of surgery are largely unknown. It is important that all conservative measures are exhausted before surgery. Since it is unlikely to help the pain, limited surgery, except total knee replacement, is contraindicated by severe degenerative changes of the patellar space. Total knee replacements (TKAs) are done often and are almost as successful as total hip replacements. Osteoarthritis is the most common reason for knee replacement.

Low Back Pain

Low back pain (LBP) affects almost one-third of the American population. Each American has an 80-percent chance of developing back pain during their lifetime. For people under the age of forty-five, problems of the back and spine are the most frequent cause of limited activity and loss of work-time.

Spinal Column

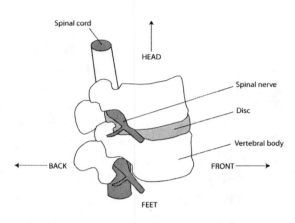

The common cold is the only disorder that occurs more frequently than low back pain. It is estimated that more than twenty-five billion dollars is spent annually in the United States during the treatment and compensation of low back injuries.

Most people feel better within a few months of the onset of acute back pain. An unfortunate 20 percent have persistent pain and future difficulties working or participating in the activities they enjoy. Much remains to be learned about each and every cause of back pain. For the most part, back pain is a result of nonspecific muscle and ligamentous strain and will resolve with conservative treatment including rest, rather than spinal surgery.

Less than 1 percent of the patients with acute low back pain have true sciatica. Most arthritis of the spine is degenerative and increases with age or follows

injuries. In ankylosing spondylitis, there is gradual fusion of the vertebral bodies of the spine over many years. This occurs in an ascending manner, starting in the low back and then ascending to the neck. The patient is usually young and has marked early morning stiffness, which improves with activity.

Rheumatoid arthritis rarely involves the lumbar spine, but it can affect the upper cervical spine. Other forms of arthritis affect the spine in one way or another. Degenerative changes cause pain with activity. Acute vertebral fractures secondary to osteoporosis resolve slowly like any other fracture, but further fractures occur if no interventions for the osteoporosis are initiated.

Disc and Facet Joint

The back is composed of the spine, muscles, ligaments, and tendons that support it. The entire structure protects the spinal cord and nerves that exit the spine at different levels. The anatomy of the spine is complex. Vertebrae stack on each other. Each vertebral body rests upon the lower one. Discs act as shock absorbers between the vertebrae. The discs are subject to all the movements of the spine. Discs protect the spine from excessive motion; however, with aging the disc slowly dries out and degenerates. As the disc degenerates, the cushioning properties are lost. The disc moves or ruptures. Movement of the disc compromises the spinal canal and presses on the spinal cord or the exiting spinal nerves branching off at each spinal level.

The vertebrae overlap with the adjacent vertebrae to form facet joints. These joints allow the spine to remain flexible in multiple directions of motion. Facet joints are a source of localized back pain as they degenerate. Obesity aggravates facet arthritis and precipitates low back pain. As OA develops with age, the joints and disc spaces develop spurs (osteophytes) that compromise the spinal canal space and press on the spinal cord. At the tiny neuroforamen exits, the nerves are pinched by the disc, bone spurs, or the combination of both and cause severe burning, hot, or piercing pain down an extremity (sciatica). The osteophytes seen on the x-ray are not the source of back pain, but are markers of the process associated with the development of OA of the spine. Surgery relieves the pressure on the nerves.

Spinal stenosis occurs when the degenerative changes compromise the central spinal canal and the required space for the spinal cord. The combination of spurs, disc herniation, or disc fragmentation encroaches on the space for the spinal cord and causes pain. Spinal stenosis of the cervical or lumbar spine requires a laminectomy to decompress the space and relieve nerve pain. Symptoms of lumbar spinal stenosis are vague and poorly localized. Leg pain on both sides is associated with numbness and weakness. The pain worsens with exer-cise and improves after short periods of rest. Symptoms are described as numbness, achy back or leg pain, a tingling or burning sensation, and buckling of the legs. Cervical spinal stenosis is associated with radiation of pain down the arms like electric shocks (parathesias), headache, and neck pain.

Shoulder

The shoulder is very different from other joints. The shoulder is non-weight bearing. The range of motion, strength, and function of both shoulders is unique. Unlike the ball and socket joint of the hip, the shoulder socket is shallow. The shoulder is like a golf ball set up on a tee rather than nestling in a deep socket like the hip. The shoulder is subject to trauma and injury daily. Areas of inflammation include the bursa, tendons, or joint. The rotator cuff is a group of muscles surrounding the shoulder. These muscles maintain stability of the joint but are often subject to injury, degeneration, and tears. Tears are painful and restrict motion at the shoulder. A tear of the rotator cuff is detected by ultrasound, arthrography, or preferably by magnetic resonance imaging (MRI). Tears of the rotator cuff are initially treated conservatively. Oral NSAIDs, physical therapy, and occasional intra-articular corticosteroids are all helpful. However, only surgery repairs a tear.

Injury and pain at the shoulder results in contraction and tightening of the muscles and other tissues around the shoulder. Bursitis or any cause of pain at the shoulder quickly results in loss of shoulder motion (adhesive capsulitis). Within a few days, individuals can't reach behind the back to fasten their clothes, put on a coat, or place their hand in the back pocket of their pants.

Total shoulder replacement or arthroplasty is most often done due to arthritis, in older individuals usually as a result of OA and in younger individuals as a result of RA. A shoulder arthroplasty is effective in relieving pain and restoring functional mobility, but not to the degree and success of other joint replacements like the hip or knee. Fusion of the shoulder joint relieves pain at the cost of mobility and is most always avoided.

Wrist

Several unique problems occur at the wrist. Carpal tunnel syndrome (CTS) is common and occurs at any age. Patients with CTS describe tingling (paresthesias) in the distribution of the median nerve, often worse at night. Carpal tunnel syndrome is associated with other conditions besides arthritis, including pregnancy, hypothyroidism, or diabetes. It occurs more commonly in women than in men. Work-related activities, especially vibratory or repetitive actions like carpentry, supermarket checking, and meat, fish, and

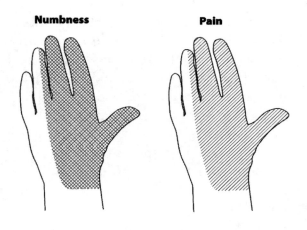

Distribution of Symptoms of Carpal Tunnel Syndrome

Numbness   Pain

poultry processing, are associated with CTS. Any inflammatory arthritis can cause CTS, but so can OA. Both hands become involved. Symptoms come on slowly and are intermittent, although they gradually occur more often and eventually are persistent. Difficulty with simple tasks like reaching for a milk carton or buttoning a shirt occurs. Late in this condition, the muscles of the thenar eminence of the thumb atrophy and become weak. These changes are irreversible.

Carpal tunnel syndrome occurs as a result of pressure on the median nerve as the nerve passes through the carpal tunnel on the inside (volar) surface of the wrist. A ligament across the wrist covers the bones from the thumb side to the little finger and forms an arch or tunnel that allows passage of the nerves, arteries, and veins to the fingers. Anything occupying the space results in pressure on the nerve. Pressure on the nerve causes pain, tingling, and eventually irreversible muscle atrophy. The tingling sensation and numbness occurs in the thumb, index finger, middle finger, and at least part of the ring finger. Without a healthy nerve, the muscles innervated by the median nerve atrophy and the handgrip is weak.

Sensory Distribution of the Median Nerve

The symptoms of CTS are often worse at night, particularly while sleeping. Individuals wake up with their hands asleep, shaking or rubbing them to bring the feeling back. There are several ways to determine if symptoms are the result of CTS. Often, it is obvious to the physician, and treatment can be undertaken without diagnostic testing. Gentle tapping over the median nerve at the area of the carpal tunnel on the volar side of the wrist will duplicate the symptoms (Tinel's sign). Holding both hands against each other in flexion or extension for several seconds will duplicate the symptoms (Phalen's sign). Many people notice the symptoms while their hands are on the steering wheel as they drive a car.

Measuring the electrical impulse of the median nerve is done by checking nerve conduction velocities (NCVs). The test is useful if surgery is contemplated and the diagnosis must be confirmed. Small needles are inserted on both sides of the wrist. A small electrical shock is sent across the wrist and measured. If there is a nerve block, the velocity of the electrical impulse is diminished. The NCV is well tolerated. NCVs are usually done by neurologists or physiatrists. Laboratory testing for other medical conditions like RA, diabetes, or hypothyroidism are useful.

Treatment for CTS should be conservative and simple. Initially, changing work activities helps. Rest periods, alternating tasks, or modifying jobs may resolve the problem. Wearing a protective splint from the drugstore at work or at night is helpful. The splint protects from excessive motion at the wrist and places the wrist in a comfortable resting position. If inflammation is a major part of the cause, a local steroid injection into the carpal tunnel space near the nerve is helpful. Oral anti-inflammatories reduce the swelling and increased pressure within the carpal tunnel space. Symptoms occurring during pregnancy will resolve after delivery. Thyroid replacement will benefit people with low thyroid and symptoms of CTS.

The symptoms of CTS may continue for years. Persistent symptoms result in irreversible weakness of the hand. Early symptoms resolve on occasion, but as time goes on the symptoms are more constant and severe. After conservative therapy or modification of activities, surgery is necessary to avoid permanent damage to the nerve. During a carpal tunnel release the surgeon cuts the ligament trapping the median nerve and the pressure on the nerve is relieved. A carpal tunnel release is an outpatient procedure. New surgical techniques now utilize a scope or laser therapy and avoid a large incision of the skin. Recovery is complete and rapid and allows the individual to return to usual activities after a few weeks. Although both wrists may have to be released, second surgeries for CTS are unusual. The treatment of carpal tunnel symptoms is summarized into a list.

Treatment of Carpal Tunnel Syndrome
◊ cock-up wrist splints
◊ change or stop repetitive activities
◊ anti-inflammatories
◊ steroid injection into the carpal tunnel
◊ surgical release

Hand

Early RA findings of the hand include swelling of the wrist, metacarpal phalangeal joints (MCPs), and the proximal interphalangeal joints (PIPs). As the arthritis progresses, subluxation at the metacarpal phalangeal joints (MCPs) and ulnar deviation occur. Subluxation of the interphalangeal joint

(IP) of the thumb causes a Z shaped deformity and interferes with pinch. The small muscles of the hand atrophy and tendons become easily visible. Characteristic changes of OA include nodal formation at the distal interphalangeal joints (DIPs) and PIPs. Squaring off at the base of the thumb at the carpal metacarpal phalangeal joint is visible. The tophi of gout occur on the fingers and other parts of the hand and exude white chalky urate crystals.

Tenosynovitis or tendinitis at the hand or wrist is common. Trigger fingers are common and are often mistaken for arthritis. The flexor tendons in the palm of the hand develop nodules. The tendons run through a sheath and a tender nodule is trapped under the sheath. The trapped tendon causes the finger to stick or trigger (trigger finger). Local corticosteroid injections of the peritendon area are particularly useful for trigger fingers. Occasionally, surgical release of the tendon is required.

CHAPTER SIXTEEN

Other Problems in Rheumatic Illness

Antiphospholipid Syndrome

The combination of increased thrombosis, miscarriages, and low platelet counts describes the antiphospholipid antibody syndrome (APL). This syndrome was first described in lupus patients. Fifty percent of patients with these antibodies do not have lupus. Studies suggest that the presence of antiphospholipid antibodies increase the future risk of deep venous thrombosis, stroke, gangrene, and heart attack. Antiphospholipid antibodies are easily detectable. There are several different antiphospholipid antibodies including the lupus anticoagulant and anticardiolipin antibody. These antibodies react with phospholipid, a fat molecule that is part of a normal cell membrane. This phenomenon causes some people to develop a false positive test for syphilis, even though they have never had the disease. Aspirin prophylaxis and even oral anticoagulants are sometimes required on a chronic basis.

Raynaud's Phenomenon

About 10 percent of the general population has Raynaud's phenomenon (RP). Only a small percentage of RP patients will develop a connective tissue disease. The diagnosis of RP is based on observation. RP is most prominent in about one third of scleroderma patients, but also occurs in individuals without any other medical problems. Blood vessels go into spasm and slow blood flow. This causes characteristic color changes of the hand or fingers. The skin feels cold. As the finger is deprived of blood it turns white and as the blood pools, the finger becomes blue or cyanotic. After the blood vessel opens up again, the skin turns red and painful. RP occurs over a few moments or longer. It involves one finger, all the fingers, or other organ parts. It is precipitated by emotions and cold, including a cool room, and is severely aggravated by smoking. It usually does not result in any tissue damage, unless associated with more serious blood vessel problems. Raynaud's phenomenon is more a nuisance than anything else, although it can be quite alarming in appearance.

Several treatment remedies are used to alleviate symptoms or lessen frequency. Mild uncomplicated RP is usually easy to control. Abstinence from smoking is mandatory. Any offending drugs should be discontinued. Avoidance of cold and abrupt changes in temperature is necessary. Insulated gloves or hand warmers are helpful. Avoidance of outdoor winter activities or cool air-conditioned rooms helps. Some antihypertensives like amlodipine (Norvasc 5 milligrams/daily) opens blood vessels and blood flow to the fingers. Although unusual, finger ulcers require significant interventions when blood flow is severely compromised. More aggressive treatment includes sympathetic blocks or surgery. Livido reticularis is a spectrum of similar vasospasm phenomena and results in mottling of the skin.

Reflex Sympathetic Dystrophy Syndrome

Regional complex pain syndrome was once referred to as reflex sympathetic dystrophy syndrome (RSDS). This syndrome is characterized by severe pain, temperature and color changes, and swelling of an extremity. The pain is severe and described as burning with an extreme sensitivity to touch or feel. The skin is mottled and changes temperature inappropriately. One extremity will perspire when the other extremity is cool or vice versa. If there is delay in recognition and early treatment, the extremity atrophies. The overlying skin will become tight and shiny. Contractures of the joint occur. There are no specific laboratory findings. The diagnosis is based on the clinical findings of vasomotor instability, pain, and history of injury. Treatment includes early corticosteroids and physical therapy. Later, a series of sympathetic blocks are necessary. Unfortunately, patients are left with permanent disability in the majority of cases.

Peptic Ulcer Disease

Peptic ulcer disease is more frequent in patients with arthritis than in the general population. Early symptoms of ulcer disease include nausea, heartburn, and stomach pain. Later, symptoms result from bleeding. Researchers estimate thousands of deaths a year as a result of bleeding or perforated ulcers because of traditional NSAID use in the United States. Fifty percent of ulcers induced by NSAIDs may be without symptoms and cause no pain.

A bacterial infection, Helicobacter pylori (*H. pylori*) is responsible for most peptic ulcers, regardless of whether these individuals have arthritis. Use of NSAIDs is responsible for 25 percent or more of the stomach ulcers not related to infection. *H. pylori* is a spiral-shaped bacteria that screws itself into the lining of the upper GI tract. Researchers are unclear how the bacteria is transmitted, but the diagnosis is relatively easy and the treatment effective. There are several ways to test for *H. pylori* infection, including serum antibodies and a biopsy of the stomach wall at the time of an upper endoscopy. Other diagnostic tests are still preliminary and under investigation.

H. pylori induced ulcers are generally confined to the upper small intestine, while NSAIDs ulcerate the stomach. *H. pylori* induced ulcers are symptomatic, while NSAID induced ulcers are asymptomatic. *H. pylori* infection is not a risk factor for NSAID induced ulcer disease. While taking NSAIDs, an ulcer may or may not be NSAID induced or secondary from *H. pylori* infection. Because the two types of ulcers are unrelated, treatment for one type won't help the other. Everyone with proven stomach ulcers should be tested for *H. pylori* infection and if present, treated with antibiotics.

NSAIDs work by inhibiting the enzyme cyclooxygenase (COX) and limit the production of prostaglandins (PGs). Research has demonstrated that good and bad PGs exist. The bad PGs play an important role mediating the inflammation of arthritis, but good PGs protect the lining of the stomach wall. Traditional NSAIDs inhibit all COX enzymes and all PGs. Without good PGs in the lining of the stomach wall there is risk for stomach ulceration.

Researchers have discovered there are two different COX enzymes. COX-1 is responsible for producing the housekeeping PGs that protect the stomach lining. Traditional NSAIDs block COX-1 and have been associated with bleeding stomach ulcers. COX-2 is responsible for PGs that create the inflammation and pain of arthritis. These PGs occur as a result of disease.

Activity of Cyclooxygenase Enzymes

◊ COX-1 is responsible for PGs protecting the stomach wall.
◊ COX-2 is responsible for the PGs producing inflammation.

Some NSAIDs selectively inhibit COX-2 and not COX-1. This leaves the housekeeping and protective mechanisms intact and decreases the incidence of bleeding and peptic ulcer disease. Unfortunately, selective COX-2 NSAIDs are believed to be associated with increased heart attack or stroke. This effect has resulted in a black box warning on all NSAIDs and the withdrawal of two of the selective COX-2 inhibitors.

Attempts to allow NSAIDs to be more tolerable doesn't necessarily make NSAIDs safer. Taking NSAIDs with food, in an upright position, or with water make NSAIDs more tolerable, but does not remove the effect on the COX enzymes. There is concern that covering up NSAID symptoms is dangerous and increases risk for bleeding because of continued use and a false sense of security.

When arthritis requires continued treatment with NSAIDs, and there is a prior history of peptic ulcer disease, or intolerance to NSAIDs, several actions are taken. Oral misoprostol (Cytotec) is a synthetic PG that replenishes the naturally occurring good PGs in the stomach wall. Misoprostol concomitantly with NSAIDs decreases the incidence of stomach ulcers. Side effects of misoprostol are mild and include diarrhea and abdominal pain that subsides after a few days. Combination medication (Arthrotec 50 or 75) includes the NSAID diclofenac (Voltaren) and misoprostol. Non-acetylated salicylates like salsalate (Disalcid) or choline magnesium trisalicylate (Trilisate) do not induce ulcers as often as traditional NSAIDs, but are still considered ulcerogenic. Coated enteric NSAIDs have no direct effect on the gastric mucosa, since they are absorbed farther down the GI tract. Enteric tablets do not prevent the systemic effect NSAIDs have on PGs. Food has a small beneficial effect. Finally, antacids like Mylanta or Maalox and H2-receptor blockers like ranitidine (Zantac), cimetidine (Tagamet), nizatidine (Axid), or famotidine (Pepcid) work by inhibiting acid production. These drugs do not prevent NSAID induced ulcers, but are effective in healing ulcers. Other potent acid inhibitors like the proton pump inhibitors (PPIs) omeprazole (Prilosec), rabeprazole (Aciphex), pantoprazole (Protonix), or lansoprazole (Prevacid) provide greater protection than the H2-receptor blockers.

The best treatment for prevention of stomach ulcers as a result of NSAID use is to minimize the use of NSAIDs and use alternative mild pain relievers when appropriate. Acetaminophen (Tylenol) is not ulcerogenic. Other risk factors like smoking, alcohol use, coumadin, significant illness, increasing age, and prior ulcer history increase the chance of developing ulcers and bleeding.

CHAPTER SEVENTEEN

Disability

Disability as a result of arthritis is significant. Arthritis and musculoskeletal disorders are the most prevalent major health problems in America. Arthritis affects over thirty million people aged forty-five years and older. About one-half of arthritis patients are over age sixty-five. Arthritis has a major impact on disability benefits, medical care, and work productivity. Arthritis increases in prevalence with increasing age. It is more common in women than men. As America grays, the impact of arthritis will become more important. Arthritis ranks significantly as a cause of long-term disability, medical visits, and prescription and nonprescription drug utilization. Arthritis accounts for a large number of all hospitalizations. The direct costs of arthritis medical care are estimated in billions of dollars every year. Clearly, arthritis care burdens health care. It comes as no surprise that quality of life issues of rheumatoid arthritis patients is equal to or worse than that of patients with congestive heart failure and diabetes. Unfortunately, the costs of unproven remedies rival these amounts.

Rheumatoid arthritis and OA are chronic illnesses lasting many years. Disability and pain accumulate slowly as joint destruction progresses. Most people with RA experience a lifetime of remissions and flares requiring ongoing medical supervision. The medical management of arthritis involves frequent monitoring. Therapeutic regimens produce measurable benefits, modify the disease course, and slow the progression.

Disability and Handicap

Disability is a major problem for persons with arthritis. Arthritis is responsible for marked reductions in work status and income. Over 50 percent of people with RA

Functional Classes of Disability	
Class One	Patients are normal in all their activities. They perform all usual activities of daily living without help.
Class Two	Patients are able to perform usual self-care and work activities but are limited in their recreational activities.
Class Three	Patients are limited at both work and recreational activities. They often use walkers or even wheelchairs.
Class Four	Patients are bedridden and limited while performing usual self-care. This level of function is serious and usually coincides with other medical problems. These patients are dependent on others for most of their basic needs and put tremendous demands on family and relatives.

lose their employment after the disease occurs. As a group, people with RA earn only 50 percent of the income expected based on age and educational level. On this basis, disability has been established as one of the greatest problems facing people with arthritis.

The Americans with Disabilities Act

The Americans with Disabilities Act (ADA) became law in 1990 and is responsible for many changes. It prohibits discrimination against persons with disabilities in employment, transportation, public accommodations, telecommunications, and services provided by the state and local government. Millions of people with arthritis are among those who benefit from

this law. Disability related to arthritis encompasses not only those who use wheelchairs or canes and crutches, but also those whose disease leads to severe fatigue, limitations of movement, pain, or loss of strength.

Functional Classification

Arthritis patients are often classified based on their ability to perform self-care activities including dressing, feeding, bathing, grooming, and toileting. Avocational activities include recreational or leisure time activities, while vocational activities include work, school, or homemaking. Function becomes a measurement of disease activity, a determination of prognosis, and a tool to determine the need for other interventions, treatment, or benefits like disability. Deterioration from one class to another in terms of needs, dependency, or reliance on others is a poor sign.

Nearly 20 percent of rheumatoid arthritis patients will stop working within one year of disease onset, 30 percent are disabled from work within five years, and 50 percent by ten years. Within one year of diagnosis, most patients with rheumatoid arthritis change their work conditions in ways such as reducing work hours, actually changing jobs, or making physical adjustments at the work place within one year of diagnosis. Once individuals leave the work force because of arthritis, they rarely return.

CHAPTER EIGHTEEN

Fact versus Myth

The facts are often difficult to sort out. The truth about arthritis is not easy to learn. Many statements are not always correct. Much of the information about arthritis is handed down from generation to generation without any objective scientific evidence. Today's access to information from the Internet makes claims of unproven remedies easily accessible and sometimes believable. Providing correct and accurate information to the patient is as important as providing medicine.

Weather and Pain

The effect the weather and climate have on arthritis is complex. It may not be weather changes that aggravate arthritis, but the stress weather causes. Studies of the effects of weather indicate symptoms worsen when the barometric pressure or humidity changes. Although a warmer and drier climate feels better, there is no scientific evidence that it will halt the disease. Some of the largest arthritis clinics in the country are in the warmest places.

Menopause

The effects of menopause are of concern for older women. Most women experience hot flashes, but fewer than half of these women are bothered enough to do anything about it. Short-term low-dose hormone replacement therapy is a reasonable option for women with severe vasomotor symptoms. Since recent concerns about estrogen and the risk for breast cancer, stroke, or heart disease, many women have discontinued estrogen replacement therapy after menopause. It is important that postmenopausal women exercise, refrain from smoking, take supplements like calcium and multivitamins, and carefully monitor their bone density for evidence of osteoporosis.

Stress

Stress does not cause arthritis and eliminating it will not end the disease. However, the impact of stress has a negative effect. Arthritis is made worse by reactions to stress. Reactions vary from individual to individual. Stress affects the ability to maintain a schedule, keep appointments, work, keep special interpersonal relationships, and continue medications on a schedule. All these factors adversely affect arthritis.

Overdoing

Too much exercise increases the pain of arthritis. Pain following exercise is a signal to take it easier. Sedentary lifestyles lead to increased stiffness. "Use it or lose it" should be embedded in the mind of patients. A joint must be moved daily to maintain range of motion. There should be a balance between exercise and inactivity or rest. During a flare of arthritis, rest is important. Stretching before and after exercise prevents stiff achy days following exercise.

Flares

A flare will not last forever, but the pain associated with exacerbations of arthritis is unbearable. Flares and remis-

sions characterize the natural course of most inflammatory arthritis. One flare should not precipitate an immediate change in drug therapy. Trends of increasing flares or other worsening parameters are a better signal that the activity of the arthritis is not responding to current therapy.

Total Hip Replacement

Total hip replacement (THR) is one of the greatest success stories of modern medicine. Since the procedure was first introduced to Americans more than twenty-five years ago, almost one million have been done. Cementing techniques have improved, complications such as infection and mechanical loosening have decreased significantly, and the rates of revision have declined. Americans undergo 300,000 THRs annually. THR is done in those people experiencing moderate to severe pain. Overall outcomes from THR are very good and getting better. Newer techniques have shortened hospital stays and lessened complications. New hip prostheses function well for twenty years or more in 80 percent of patients. Failure rates are extremely low.

Drugs over the Counter

Several years ago, the Food and Drug Administration (FDA) began approving nonprescription strength of popular anti-inflammatory medications only previously prescribed. These medications are now available on both sides of the counter, by prescription in higher doses and over the counter (OTC) in lower doses. Some medications have moved exclusively to the OTC status. The trend appears unlikely to abate and the future of self-medication seems bright. The pharmaceutical industry obviously supports these OTC switches with high hopes.

When prescription medications go OTC, they are much more available. Consumers do not need to see a physician or pharmacist to obtain medications. When a drug goes OTC, sales goes up quickly. In the crusade against rising health care costs, self-medication represents one of the least costly components of health care expenditures. Consumer insurance plans cover prescription medications, but not OTCs. This results in more out-of-pocket expenses for the patient. It is argued that because the OTCs cost less and are paid for by the patient, health insurance dollars are saved. Saving health insurance dollars keeps health insurance premiums lower to the consumer.

One significant risk of OTCs is taking medications for seemingly minor symptoms that are really signs of more serious disease. As a precaution, the FDA has typically recommended lower dosages and label warnings about side effects and symptoms.

Liver Biopsy

Liver biopsy remains the gold stan-dard for detection of cirrhosis, but the decision whether to perform a biopsy in MTX treated RA patients is difficult. The risk of developing MTX induced cirrhosis is uncertain, the natural history of the liver disease is unknown, and there are no reliable clinical laboratory findings to guide the physician in the decision when to do a liver biopsy. With the increasing use of MTX as a long-term therapy in RA, this issue is of great importance. Few liver biopsies will be done in the future for MTX toxicity because alternative treatment choices exist and it is not necessary to continue MTX in all patients.

Collagen

Collagen is a substance made of protein that supports various structures throughout the body. It is the most important component of connective tissue found in blood vessels, skin, joints, kidneys, heart, and lung. Diseases affecting many of these organ systems are referred to as connective tissue diseases or collagen vascular diseases. These same diseases are autoimmune illnesses. Supplemental oral collagen sources (chicken cartilage) remain an unproven remedy for arthritis.

Early Arthritis

Early diagnosis of different rheumatic diseases is difficult because of the similar clinical manifestations among them. A symmetrical arthritis of small and medium sized joints is the first symptom in rheumatoid arthritis, polymyositis, lupus, scleroderma, and other rheumatic illnesses. Rheumatic illnesses can evolve into overlap syndromes, appearing like more than one rheumatic illness or changing characteristics to resemble a different connective tissue disease entirely. Not until rheumatic disorders develop into a definitive arthritis is diagnosis, treatment, and prognosis absolutely determined.

The earlier DMARDs are started in RA, the less structural joint changes are likely to occur. A small percentage of patients with an early rheumatic illness like RA will have a short-lived and self-limiting illness. It is reasonable to not start a DMARD until disease appears persistent and the diagnosis is confirmed over at least a few weeks or months after the onset.

Diet and More

Researchers have continually tried to determine how and why diet influences the course of arthritis. Since arthritis is generally a lifelong disease, it is not surprising that researchers and patients seek out a role food may play in arthritis. It is not clear to what extent foods affect the symptoms of arthritis. Eating a well-balanced diet to maintain energy and strength is as important for people with arthritis as it is for anyone else. Overweight people should lose weight to reduce the amount of stress on sore joints. While dietary manipulation may be useful in the management of common medical conditions like heart disease or diabetes, it is much less accepted in the management of arthritis. Research has shown that only a small percent of people with RA flare after eating a specific food. If there is a specific food that does seem to aggravate arthritis, it should be avoided or eliminated from the diet. Currently, there is no special food that must be eliminated or added to the diets of people with arthritis.

Omega-3 fatty acids and antioxidants prevent inflammation. Omega-3 fatty acids are found in cold-water fish like tuna, salmon, herring, sardines, and mackerel. Other foods rich in omega-3 fatty acids include beans, flax, green leafy vegetables, and olive oil. Potential obstacles to fish oil supplements include the expense, a fishy taste, or large daily quantities of the capsules required. The onset of action of fish oil is delayed with effects being evident at about twelve weeks. There is very little evidence that supplementation with antioxidants such as vitamin E, C, and selenium provide significant clinical improvement. Tea contains antioxidants, which helps inhibit prostaglandins and possibly inflammation. A diet rich in antioxidants counteracts free-oxygen radicals produced by inflammatory cells. It is best to get these compounds in the diet and food, rather than supplements. Until we know more, it is still adequate for arthritis patients to eat a well-balanced diet, maintain weight, and exercise.

Potatoes, eggplant, tomatoes, and green peppers all belong to the same family of plants (nightshades). Many people believe that eating from this group leads to a buildup of toxins that aggravates arthritis. There is no evidence that this is true and avoiding these foods can diminish a good source of vitamin C. Exclusion diets help only a small minority of arthritis patients. Allergenic foods supposedly reduce arthritis because they are arthrogenic.

The risk of gout increases with the consumption of meat and seafood, but decreases with the consumption of low-fat dairy products. The mechanism remains to be determined.

A placebo response or psychological factor may contribute to the improvements seen in arthritis patients who change their diet. Malnutrition can suppress the immune system and benefit an inflammatory arthritis. A change in gut flora as a result of a change in diet may alter the array of bacteria present in the bowel, diminish the absorption of foreign bacterial proteins through the bowel wall, and promote a subsequent response by the immune system.

Finally, oral tolerization, or the ingestion of small amounts of a foreign protein like collagen (chicken cartilage), has never shown significant efficacy in the treatment of inflammatory arthritis.

Chondroprotective

The term chondroprotective is deceiving. A chondroprotective treatment retards, arrests, or even reverses disease of cartilage. It is suggested that some medications are chondroprotective. It is unfortunate that this term is used in advertising and gives false impressions about the benefits of treatment that are not realistic at this time. No known treatment is currently chondroprotective.

Knuckle-Cracking

Cracking knuckles has no health benefits and causes no known long-term problems. The cracking sounds a joint makes when it is stretched, pushed, or pulled are caused by pressure within the joint capsule. Knuckle cracking does not lead to any type of arthritis or joint degeneration. Instead, it is an annoying habit.

Depression: Not Necessarily Part of the Disease

Depression occurs frequently during the course of arthritis. There is often uncertainty as to whether or not it is to be expected because of the stresses of the illness. States of depression are induced by the disease, by various medications used to treat arthritis, or by countless other factors in one's life. Depression is not to be confused with the everyday experiences of a mild mood swing

Symptoms of Depression	
Psychological	**Physical**
◊ sadness and gloom	◊ headache
◊ crying without provocation	◊ palpitations
◊ insomnia or restless sleep	◊ diminished sexual interest
◊ loss of appetite or overeating	◊ body aches, pain
◊ uneasiness or anxiety	◊ indigestion
◊ irritability	◊ constipation
◊ feelings of guilt or remorse	◊ diarrhea
◊ lowered self-esteem	
◊ inability to concentrate	
◊ poor memory and recall	
◊ indecisiveness	
◊ lack of interest	
◊ fatigue	

that everyone experiences during difficult times. On the other hand, a serious depression is disabling, unpleasant, and prolonged. A variety of physical and psychological symptoms occur.

Just a few of these symptoms are enough to seriously disrupt life. Important symptoms are sense of failure, loss of social interest, sense of punishment, suicidal thoughts, dissatisfaction, indecision, and crying. People who feel hopeless believe that their distressing symptoms will never get better. People who feel helpless think they are beyond help and no one cares enough to help them or could succeed in helping, even if they tried. Many of the symptoms of depression go unrecognized in a chronic disease like arthritis.

Symptoms are similar to those of the underlying medical condition. Even when recognized, depression goes untreated or inadequately treated.

Denial of arthritis interferes with early recognition, early treatment, and early relief of symptoms. Life with arthritis requires a series of adaptations and adjustments and each poses its own set of challenges. The need to develop new skills becomes important. It becomes necessary to focus on one success at a time, so that a pattern of success occurs more often than failure.

Survival

Studies in the long-term outcome of

rheumatic disease generally emphasize functional status, work disability, and the reduction of quality of life, rather than survival or mortality. Yet patients often ask during the course of disease if they will die of their arthritis. The cause of death in individuals with rheumatic disease is often not recognized as rheumatic illness. Documentation on death certificates usually includes diagnoses like acute stroke or heart disease. The more serious rheumatic diseases with higher death rates or mortality are rare, including SLE, vasculitis, or scleroderma.

Nonetheless, it is recognized that higher mortality rates are seen in arthritis and most rheumatic illness in than the population without arthritis. Higher death rates are associated with more severe disease. For example, SLE nephritis has one of the poorest responses of any disease and is associated with increased mortality rates. During the past several years, there has been significant improvement because of increased disease recognition, more sensitive diagnostic tests, and treatment. Early treatment appears to improve survival. Death should not be considered unrelated to the arthritis. Rheumatic disease is considered a predisposing risk factor for infection, cardiovascular disease, or other conditions to which death is attributed.

Osteoarthritis appears to be associated with higher death rates, although the rates are modest compared to the other inflammatory rheumatic illnesses. Even so, because OA is the most common rheumatic illness, higher mortality rates become an important health problem in the general population.

It is clearly understood that patients with RA die at an age earlier than would be expected for individuals of the same age and sex in the general population. It is rarely mentioned as cause of death, yet RA is associated with an average seven-year reduction of survival. There is a general underestimation of the mortality in RA. Patients with RA who are at risk of early mortality are identified by evidence of more severe systemic disease. Death is rarely explained by drug toxicity or other treatments.

Because of the predisposition to higher mortality rates among patients with rheumatic diseases, the argument is made that specialty medical care is both cost-effective and ethical in the long-term strategy for arthritis patients.

Pregnancy's Effects on Arthritis

There is something very different about the immune system in pregnancy. Pregnancy alters the expression of the connective tissue diseases and results in some improvement or worsening of symptoms. There is no doubt that sex hormones influence the immune system. Most connective tissue diseases are more common in women than men. The incidence of RA has a three-to-one ratio of women to men, while lupus is nine to one. Lupus is much more common during the childbearing years.

Many patients with RA experience relief of symptoms during their third trimester of pregnancy. Improvement with contraceptives or estrogens encourages some alternative clinics to treat with estrogens, even though this remains to be proven or accepted as standard therapy.

During pregnancy, lupus patients improve, stay the same, or even worsen. Lupus patients have no difficulty getting pregnant. Instead, the problem is staying pregnant and carrying a fetus to term safely. It is important that the disease is quiescent at the time of conception and pregnant women not take fetal toxic drugs or expect to need fetal toxic drugs during pregnancy. Antiphospholipid antibodies are responsible for fetal loss, low birth weights, stillbirth, and miscarriage in lupus patients. These antibodies predispose to blood clots in the placenta.

Pill Splitting Is OK

One solution to the high cost of prescription medication is to split the higher dosage of medication into two pieces. Many medications, regardless of the dose, are priced similarly. Splitting the higher dosed pill will effectively cut the price in half. For the millions of Americans uninsured for prescription medications, pill splitting provides a significant cost savings. Many medications split safely without too much difficulty. Some medications are not candidates for splitting, including time-released

medications and capsules. Even with pill splitting devices, splitting medications can result in dose variation. The decision to split pills is best made between physician and patient after carefully considering safety issues. Switching to a generic medicine or alternative drug therapy might be more appropriate.

CHAPTER NINETEEN

Joint Surgery

Surgery plays a role for those individuals experiencing unacceptable pain or limitation of function due to structural joint damage. Whether inflammation of the joints is successfully controlled or eliminated, patients may have already experienced significant joint damage. The most successful surgical procedures include carpal tunnel release at the wrist, resection of the heads of the metatarsal bones of the foot, joint replacement of the metacarpal phalangeal joints, and total hip or knee replacements. For most patients with arthritis, surgery will never be necessary.

Most arthritis is controlled with conservative management including medication, physical or occupational therapy, exercise, and rest. Arthritis cannot be cured by surgery. In addition, consideration must be given to operating on one or a few joints in a disease that affects many at one time. The question must be asked whether the stress of surgery and the postoperative period is worth the results. In some cases, this is difficult to decide and in others, it is easy. The decision to have surgery is a serious one and should never be taken lightly. Patients should be well informed, educated, and aware of other options or alternative treatments to surgery. Second opinions from other surgeons are reasonable, if the second surgeon is provided all the available medical records, x-rays, laboratory tests, and is allowed to reexamine the patient.

Orthopedic Surgeon

It is important that the patient and family have realistic expectations about the outcome of the surgery, both in respect to appearance and function, but also potential complications and post-surgical needs including physical therapy, extra help at home, and medications for pain control. The rheumatologist should orchestrate the timing of surgery in arthritis patients because of the complexity of the issues. The orthopedic surgeon explains the procedure, risks, and benefits of surgery.

It is not uncommon that individuals with arthritis need several surgeries. Prior to surgery, there are special needs for medications, extra corticosteroid doses, or the need to stop medications that aggravate bleeding.

Cartilage Repair

Damaged cartilage results in arthritis. The best treatment is to repair the damage or replace the cartilage. Modern medicine hasn't discovered how to repair injured or diseased cartilage entirely. Surgery repairs or removes damaged cartilage in order to prevent further destruction of the joint, lessen pain, and improve motion. Cartilage repair must overcome several challenges before it is universally successful.

Abrasion arthroplasty removes frayed fragments of cartilage. Abrasion arthroplasty removes diseased hyaline cartilage and allows the regeneration of fibrocartilage. Shaving the irregular surface improves the unnecessary friction and mechanical symptoms of unstable fragments at the margins of the cartilage. During debridement, the joint is lavaged and flooded with large volumes of fluid. The lavage removes cartilage debris and many chemical mediators of inflammation in the joint fluid. Abrasion arthroplasty provides some symptomatic pain relief. The abrasion of damaged cartilage and exposure of the underlying

bone creates bleeding and brings new cells to the area. The scar that occurs is fibrocartilage and is of uncertain durability compared to the original hyaline cartilage that covered the bone. At least one well-publicized medical study suggested there was no difference at all after arthroscopy if the joint was lavaged, debrided, or had nothing done at all. Regardless of the initial pain relief, current belief is that the benefits of arthroscopy alone rapidly decline with time.

Surgeons attempt to stimulate new cartilage growth over the end of bones by drilling and creating small micro fractures on the surface of the cartilage. The micro fractures are intended to bring cells to grow new cartilage. The new cartilage formed is unfortunately subject to accelerated degeneration. The formation of fibrocartilage is not as suitable to bearing weight as the hyaline cartilage.

Cartilage tissue implantation has the potential to repair cartilage. Various tissue implantation techniques have been explored. It is possible to remove a small number of cartilage cells from a normal area of cartilage and grow these cells in the laboratory. Later, a localized area of injured cartilage is debrided and the patient's own cells inserted into the defect. This tissue implantation (autologous) holds promise, but is still in its infancy. The procedure is done in large medical centers equipped to grow the cells and monitor the benefits. Osteochondral grafts are used to fill defects of normal cartilage. Although results are encouraging, the transplantation of small plugs taken from a nearby donor site of the same patient has the same limitations of other repair procedures. Grafts taken from cadavers (allograft) are used to fill large defects. Since rejections are unusual, tissue typing is not necessary. The cartilage's poor blood supply doesn't allow cartilage the ability to reject the graft. There is a risk of disease transmission with this type of tissue transplantation. Current research of cartilage repair focuses on biogradeable polymers. The polymers act as the scaffolding to hold transplanted cartilage cells and stimulate cell growth. It is likely that this type of therapeutic approach will play an important role in the future of cartilage restoration.

Indications for Surgery

Although the primary indications for surgery are either improved function or relief of pain, evaluating the need for surgery is difficult. To operate for pain relief is sometimes a difficult decision. Pain at night (nocturnal pain) is often a clear-cut indication for joint replacement in hip disease.

Arthroscopy

Arthroscopy provides access into the joint. Originally used in large joints like the knee, arthroscopes are now used in almost all joints. The procedure is typically done on an outpatient basis under general or regional anesthesia. Complications of arthroscopy are unusual, but are related to bleeding, the introduction of foreign material, or immobility, thrombophlebitis, infection, or compressive neuropathy. The advantages as compared to arthrotomy include a shortened recovery period, earlier mobility, and less cost compared to a prolonged stay in the hospital.

Recent criticism has suggested that some arthroscopies are unnecessary and the benefits questionable. In older adults, MRI findings may suggest a torn meniscus, which is really representative of arthritis, especially at the knee. Repairing this meniscus is not as beneficial to an older adult as compared to the young athlete with an acute injury and pain. Following an injury, a torn meniscus creates mechanical pains that are relieved by resection of the torn fragments of the cartilage. In older individuals without a history of specific injury, the torn meniscus may not be the only source of knee pain. Resection of the meniscus will not relieve pain in these older individuals. It is interesting to look inside the joint and remove joint debris, but the benefits to the patient are limited.

Synovectomy

During a synovectomy, the orthopedic surgeon removes the inflammatory synovial cells in and around the joint, including the sheath around tendons next to the joint. Synovectomy is done to prevent further damage to the tendon and joint surface. The articular surfaces are left intact and preserved. The popularity of synovectomy has declined compared to past years when this surgery was more in favor. Regardless, synovectomy is still appropriate on occasion and provides palliative relief for years in those individuals with disease limited to a just a few joints. The inflammatory synovium around a tendon are removed surgically for the relief of triggering or other dysfunction of the tendons. On occasion, as much can be achieved by injecting corticosteroids. Tendon rupture requires repair in addition to removal of the inflammatory synovium.

Resection Arthroplasty

Resection arthroplasty removes a portion of an otherwise damaged joint. This is done when the joint is not necessary for weight bearing. Arthrodesis, or joint fusion, alleviates pain at the joint at the sacrifice of motion. It should be avoided if possible, but in some cases there is no choice. Fusion of the carpal metacarpal phalangeal joint of the thumb is useful and allows improved function when instability of that joint interferes with a strong pinch.

Joint Replacements

Joint replacement or reconstructive surgery creates a permanent change to the joint. Joint replacement is considered in those individuals after severe permanent changes of the cartilage occur, the x-ray shows severe joint space narrowing, and the physical exam reveals crepitation, pain, swelling, and limited range of motion. Total joint replacement has revolutionized the care of all arthritis patients.

Concern centers around the durability of the prosthesis. Revision of total joint replacements is possible, but difficult. Durability is limited because of loosening or the occurrence of infection. Loosening is determined by x-ray. A painful joint implant requires aspiration and removal of fluid to examine for infection. Infection usually requires removal of the prosthesis and a prolonged period of immobility. The patient is functionally without a joint. Removal of a total hip replacement only allows the patient to ambulate on crutches, while the removal of a total knee replacement limits the patient to transferring from bed to chair. Following the initial removal of the infected prosthesis, prolonged intravenous antibiotics are given before a second prosthesis is inserted.

Total joint replacement provides prompt pain relief. Postoperative pain resolves with time. The replacement of the shoulder joint has unique challenges for the patient and surgeon. Patients with severe RA will invariably have significant deterioration of the rotator cuff and muscles around the shoulder. This often precedes advanced destruction of the articular cartilage. Disuse of the shoulder muscles adds to weakness and limited range of motion. In RA, shoulder replacement does not always result in as good a range of motion as anticipated. This argues for seeking a shoulder joint replacement early in RA.

Bloodless Surgery

Bloodless surgery programs are established to meet the demands for surgical treatment without the use of donor blood or stored blood. Religious and personal reasons are justifiable reasons for not wanting a blood transfusion. Objectives of bloodless strategies are to utilize all available resources to minimize blood loss. Techniques include salvage and the reinfusion of the patient's own blood, cell-salvage techniques at the time of surgery, and treatment with drug therapy to maximize the patient's own blood production.

Joint replacement surgery often necessitates blood transfusions. Following major joint replacement, fewer blood transfusions are given now than in past years because of bloodless surgery techniques. Patients are allowed to build up their hemoglobin prior to their surgery by taking iron supplements or injections of the red cell stimulating hormone erythropoietin (Procrit, Epogen). Autologous blood transfusions or self-directed transfusions are donated several days before elective surgery and given postoperatively as needed. Cell-saver techniques allow lost blood at the time of the operation to be filtered and given back to the patient during surgery or shortly thereafter. During operations associated with significant bleeding, cell-saver techniques save large amounts of blood. Newer surgical techniques result in less bleeding at the time of surgery. Many operations routinely done through large incisions in the past are now done with small scopes percutaneously. Finally, in relatively healthy individuals, blood counts are allowed to dip lower than previously acceptable.

On occasion, transfusions are still necessary. The blood supply in America has never been safer. The risk for infection with transfusion-transmitted viruses has never been lower. Expansion of blood donor screening and improvements to laboratory markers have reduced the risk for HIV and hepatitis C infection. Despite improvements, a zero-risk blood supply does not exist.

Prosthetic Joint Infections

The use of antibiotics during the perioperative surgery time and laminar flow techniques in the operating room have reduced the risk of infection following joint replacements to less than 1 to 2 percent for hip and knee replacements. Early infections are usually abrupt and characterized by acute pain, swelling, fever, and warmth over the implanted prosthesis. Late infections present with less obvious symptoms. Once infection is identified, treatment must be prompt and specific. The goal of treatment is to relieve pain and return to a functional joint replacement. Therapies include intravenous antibiotics and on occasion surgical removal of the joint implant. At the time of surgery, the infection is drained and the area debrided of infected or necrotic tissue. If the prosthesis is removed, a second prosthesis is replaced later. Long-term antibiotics therapy is commonly used to continue to suppress infection.

The consequence of a septic joint replacement is significant. Prophylactic antibiotic therapy is given to patients with prior joint replacements whenever bacteremia occurs (dental prophylaxis).

Specialized Surgeries

New surgeries and techniques are constantly explored. Unispacer implants are inserted in the medial side of the knee joint, but these have not been as rewarding as initially hoped. The implant is a small kidney-shaped insert made of cobalt that is intended to stay in place without the use of screws or cement in individuals who put a low demand on their knee. Early enthusiasm has been blunted because of poor outcomes, including dislocation of the device. Removal of the implant leads to a total knee replacement.

New surgical approaches for total hip replacement are encouraging. It may soon be possible to do surgery in the morning with patients sleeping in their own beds that night at home. Minimally invasive total hip replacement shrinks the length of stay in the hospital to the bare essential. The procedure is technically challenging for the surgeon. A small incision avoids cutting muscles and tendons. Postoperative pain is less and the recovery much quicker. Potentially, total hip replacement will be an outpatient procedure. The rationale for smaller incisions is faster recovery. The patient and surgeon selection is key. The learning curve for the surgeon is steep. Minimally invasive total knee replacement is problematic. If arthritis changes are limited to one side of the knee joint, unicompartment (unilateral) knee replacements are much easier to do than a total knee replacement. Conversion to total knee replacement may be necessary in the future.

Timing of Surgery

Except for a few instances, surgery in the arthritis patient is elective. There are few indications for emergency operations. Immediate intervention is necessary if there is evidence to suggest instability of the cervical spine. Subluxation of the first two cervical vertebrae results in serious impingement of the spinal cord. Surgical fusion of the first two cervical vertebrae is appropriate in many RA patients with severe long-standing disease. Repairs of tendon ruptures are necessary to prevent further harm and maintain function. Drainage of a septic joint or removal of an infected prosthesis is almost always a surgical emergency.

One must understand that orthopedic surgery is only one of several options to consider in an attempt to integrate the total management and care of the arthritis patient. Important principles include the understanding that the arthritis will not be cut out by surgery and to operate for pain alone usually results in more pain. The stress of surgery aggravates other comorbid problems. The required immobility increases the potential for pneumonia, thrombophlebitis, and hospital acquired (iatrogenic) disease or illness, including blood transfusion or drug reactions.

Anticoagulation

Patients undergoing elective hip replacement or knee replacement are at risk for developing thrombophlebitis in the deep veins of the leg and pelvis. Pulmonary emboli may be large enough to cause severe respiratory distress and death or small enough not to cause symptoms. Since death secondary to pulmonary emboli often occurs on the first day of symptoms, the identification of high-risk individuals is important. Preventive anticoagulation during the high-risk period is preferred to a strategy of waiting for a blood clot in the legs to occur. Deep vein thrombophlebitis (DVT) can cause a post-thrombotic

syndrome of leg swelling, pain, and skin ulcerations.

Effective measures to prevent DVT are recommended for a minimum of seven to ten days after major orthopedic surgery. Recommended anticoagulants include injected subcutaneous heparin like enoxaparin (Lovenox) or oral warfarin (Coumadin). Extending the duration of anticoagulation therapy after surgery reduces the incidence of blood clots. The risk for blood clots continues for at least four weeks after surgery. Continuation of anticoagulation further decreases the incidence of blood clots for thirty or more days without significant risk for bleeding. Initiating anticoagulation six hours after the completion of surgery minimizes bleeding risks.

CHAPTER TWENTY

Rehabilitation and Exercise

Allied health care professionals are important in the care of the arthritis patient. Maintaining the function and productivity of patients with arthritis requires coordinated multidisciplinary care. Health care professionals include nurses, physical and occupational therapists, social workers, dietitians, educators, psychologists, and rehabilitation specialists. All these professionals offer the patient with arthritis different advice. Physical therapists demonstrate exercises to keep bones and muscles fit and strong. Occupational therapists help with activities of daily living (ADLs), especially upper extremity activities, splints, or assistive devices that can make life easier or more accessible.

Exercise

Regular exercise and physical activity are important to the health of people with arthritis. In fact, studies suggest that not exercising is risky. What may seem like very small benefits resulting from exercise and physical activity can make an impact on all aspects of life. Just about every arthritis patient can safely do some form of physical activity. Everyday physical activities accomplish some of the same goals as exercise. The key is to increase physical activity, exercise, and remain independent. Patients have to find their own way to exercise. They have to embrace it and make it work for them. Exercise helps relieve anxiety and stress and improve mood.

Strengthening Exercise

Arthritis patients lose strength. Small changes in muscle mass make a difference in strength for these patients. Gradually increasing amounts of weight are necessary for strengthening exercises. Muscle soreness and slight fatigue are normal after muscle-building exercises, but exhaustion, sore joints, and unpleasant muscle pulling are not. No exercise should cause worsening joint pain. Exercises for strength benefit balance. Stretching exercises help flexibility, but alone will not improve endurance or strength. Exercise helps maintain range-of-motion, strength, and endurance, as well as making further gains and improvements. Strong muscles and tissues around a joint support and protect an inflamed joint.

Without exercise, joints become stiff and muscles weak. The most comfortable position for a painful joint is flexion, yet prolonged flexion prevents full extension later. Extremities with fixed flexion deformities are not as strong as a normal joint with a full range of motion. When the wrist is fixed in extension, it is stronger than when the wrist is fixed in flexion. Propping a swollen painful knee over a pillow in a flexed position encourages fixed flexion deformities. Ambulating with flexion deformities is difficult and requires significant energy demands. Range-of-motion exercises are most important at the shoulder. There are few activities that put the shoulder through a full range of motion.

Arthritis patients require an individualized exercise program of range-of-motion, endurance, and strengthening exercises. All programs planned by ther-

apists should be for home or other independent activity. Therapy is not continued for extended periods (maintenance). To justify physical therapy, there is continued progressive improvement and the need for monitoring by a physical or occupational therapist.

With exercise, daily activities are easier, safer, and more enjoyable. Exercise improves overall health and fitness by increasing energy levels, sleep and rest, weight, cardiac reserve, bones and muscle strength, and improves mood, self-esteem, and a sense of well-being. Exercise prevents injury and further joint damage by making cartilage healthier.

Isometric Exercise

There are two important types of strengthening exercises. Isometric exercises tighten the muscle, but do not move the joint. This is helpful when movement of the joint hurts. Isometric exercise builds strong muscles without precipitating pain that might discourage further activities. To prevent further injury, isometric exercise stabilizes joints and provides a more even distribution of weight. Quad sets are a good isometric exercise for the knee joint. The large muscles of the anterior thigh are tightened without flexion of the knee. Quad sets are done in bed or sitting upright in a good supportive chair. The leg is held out parallel to the floor for a several seconds.

Isotonic Exercise

Isotonic exercises move the joint and build strong muscles by slowly increasing the number of repetitions or adding light weights. Pool therapy adds resistance. Benefits of the water include the buoyancy and warmth. The water supports the body and puts less stress on the larger joints. Warm water relaxes the muscles and provides immediate relief and motion. Several exercises can be done in a shallow area of a pool without swimming. The Arthritis Foundation sponsors community pool programs. Health clubs have a variety of equipment that accomplishes many of the same goals in an interesting and different way.

Endurance Exercise

Endurance exercises are beneficial to people even without arthritis. Active exercises increase energy and stamina, controls weight, and improves mood. Simple activities include walking, swimming, and biking. These exercises encourage individuals to reach specific goals, increase walking capacity, and improve daily activities. Muscle disuse from inactivity quickly erodes strength. Muscles atrophy within a few days of disuse. Muscles at complete rest shrink 3 percent daily. Gaining back strength and muscle bulk takes months to recover. Once a swollen knee improves, strengthening the quadriceps muscles decreases pain, increases function, and improves safety.

Aerobic Exercise

Aerobic exercise requires repetitive activities of large muscles intended to increase cardiovascular efficiency and improve muscular endurance and activity tolerance. Arthritis patients can successfully perform aerobic exercises without exacerbating the underlying signs and symptoms of arthritis. Walking increasingly greater distances increases funcion, and decreases arthritic pain levels in those individuals with arthritis of the knee. Aerobic activities should be specifically tailored to a patient's needs, begun slowly, and minimize symptom aggravation to maximize compliance. Common aerobic exercises include walking, stationary bicycle riding, and swimming. Since the buoyancy of the water unloads the joints, pool exercises are helpful for those individuals with weight-bearing pain.

Exercise Precautions

An exercise program is approached with care to minimize risk. Physical fitness and training declines with age. The decline is accelerated in those individuals with arthritis. Proper exercise training reverses or at least slows this process. Overloading the muscular system is known as resistance training (weight training) and is currently popular at health fitness centers. Weight training results in improved muscular strength, endurance, and recovery from the stresses imposed by physical activity and injury. The maintenance of muscle mass has been demonstrated to be increasingly important in the reduction of body fat, improvement in cardiopulmonary fitness, reduction of blood pressure, reduction of falls, and improved cholesterol profiles. In those individuals with arthritis and related conditions, resistance training increases the potential for a greater quality of life.

Weight Control with Exercise

One of the biggest reasons for the growing obesity epidemic is the fact that few people exercise. It is estimated that over one-half of American adults do not perform the minimum amount of exercise needed. Over 25 percent of adults do not perform any type of exercise. This is despite the fact that people recognize the benefits of exercise including reducing the risk for heart disease, improving blood pressure, alleviating depression, and helping arthritis. More than one third of the population is estimated to be overweight with an additional 15 percent estimated to be obese. The problem is worse in women and minorities. Incorporating exercise into a daily regime is a lifestyle change.

Heat or Cold

Therapists use different thermal modalities to provide relief to swollen and painful joints. Warmth provides a soothing and deep penetrating relief, but should be used carefully. Heat relaxes muscles and stimulates the circulation. Cold temperatures provide pain relief. Two opposite modalities like hot or cold temporarily relieve the pain and swelling of some forms of arthritis, yet neither method works for all people all the time. Some patients prefer heat, while others prefer the cold, and some do not prefer either. Yet others get relief by alternating hot and cold to a localized area. Finding the most effective treatment requires a certain amount of trial and error.

Hot and cold have distinct advantages compared to other modalities. Most hot and cold applications are readily available at home without any expense. A package of frozen peas makes an excellent ice pack. Electrical heating pads are readily available in most households. Sleeping with a heating pad for a prolonged period is dangerous and should be avoided. Heat tends to stimulate the circulation in a localized area and cold tends to numb an area and reduce inflammation. For many people with arthritis, a hot shower in the morning is all they need to loosen their stiff joints. Hot or cold should be applied in short intervals, perhaps only fifteen to twenty minutes at a time. Hot packs, hot showers or baths, rubs, or paraffin wax treatments provide superficial heating. Hot packs are moist or dry and can include mud baths, spa water, or mineral baths. Hot or cold treatments are applied only to healthy, clean, and dry skin. Open sores or cuts should be protected and checked regularly for infection. Diathermy is a physical therapy modality of deep penetrating heating. Ultrasound is the most penetrating of all heating modalities.

Transcutaneous Nerve Stimulation

Transcutaneous nerve stimulation (TENs) is a modality of pain control without oral medication. It offers pain relief through the use of a tiny electrical impulse and has been in use since the late 1960s. The body of the TENs unit houses batteries and operating controls. Electrodes are attached with small wires to adhere to the skin and placed over the area of pain. The electrodes direct a small electrical charge to the spot that produces the most effective pain control. The unit is mobile and is easily carried. The treatment area is changed from day to day for the most effective coverage of pain relief. The tingling created by the electrical stimulation blocks the brain's ability to receive pain stimulation, almost like a telephone line that can handle only one message at a time. Some believe that the electrical stimulation stimulates the brain to produce its own pain-killing chemicals. Two basic modes on the unit allow either a constant tingling sensation to block other pain signals or a pulsating charge to stimulate the brain's production of its own natural painkillers.

The reaction to a TENs unit is quite variable and individualized. Some people will achieve no benefit and others cannot function without them. Although the response differs depending on the type of pain relief sought, most patients get some pain relief. The success of TENs is dependent on the patient. The patient must experiment with the location of the electrodes and adjust the mode of current and the intensity of the charge. An experienced physical therapist monitors TENs use during a period of evaluation.

Cane

A cane is intended to offer weight support while walking. A single-point cane is for those who need a minimal degree of support and stability. A quad cane is for those individuals with limited mobility, but who need a more stable cane. A variety of handles are available for canes including a crook style, tee style, orthopedic style, or swan neck style. The handle helps to distribute the weight evenly for additional support and a comfortable grip. It is important that a cane is adjusted to the proper length. To find the proper length, the patient stands as naturally as possible on a firm and flat surface. When the handle of the cane touches the inside of the wrist where it meets the palm, the cane is the proper length. A cane is used on the less painful side. Canes are difficult to use for those patients with severe deformities or active synovitis of their wrists and fingers.

Footwear

Even without arthritis, foot pain is a common complaint. Poorly fitted shoes cause discomfort and injury. Shoe size changes with time and the ravage of arthritis. Frequent measuring of shoe size is important; however, many shoe sizes do not correspond to the expected fit. This necessitates trying on shoes and actually walking in them. The forefront of the shoe provides space for the toes. The space must be wide and deep to provide for the deformities of arthritis. The soles of the shoe should be light, flexible, and long wearing. Shoe inserts or orthotics may be necessary. There must be ample room to prevent skin ulceration.

Occupational Therapy

Like the physical therapist, the registered occupational therapist (OTR) is an important allied health care professional who deals with exercise, strengthening, range of motion, and joint protection. Joint protection lessens pain and discomfort associated with some activities and discourages deformity. There are some activities done during the day that actually increase the tendency toward deformity. Splinting an inflamed wrist at night in extension lessens the symptoms of carpal tunnel syndrome and provides for a stronger power grip. On occasion,

deformities are so severe that the OTR manufactures custom splints.

Activities of Daily Living

Occupational therapists deal with activities of daily living (ADLs), especially upper extremity activities, splints, or assistive devices that make life easier or more accessible. With a bit of ingenuity and specialized training, the OTR finds less stressful ways for the patient to do almost any activity. Placing heavy objects on lower shelves in the kitchen, a grab bar by the toilet, or a handle on the step from the garage into the house can make a world of difference for some people. Planning in advance, resting periodically, carrying smaller and fewer loads, and utilizing handles on grocery bags are helpful. Important devices suggested by the occupational therapist include: elastic shoelaces, slip-on shoes, built-up handles on pencils or eating utensils, Velcro instead of buttons, long-handled shoehorns, buttonhooks, zippers with pull rings, and more.

Work Simplification

It is important for the arthritis patient to conserve energy and make it simple. Patients learn to avoid prolonged sitting, standing, or pressure on the same joints for long periods. Sliding rather than lifting, keeping heavy objects on the lowest shelf, and using multipurpose and lightweight equipment with built-up handles if necessary makes grasping easier and safer.

Joint Protection

Joint protection avoids forces and stresses that damage joints. The force on a joint depends on the amount of weight it has to support and the length of time the movement takes. If muscles exert too much force over an inflamed joint, the tissues around the joint no longer support it or keep the muscles aligned properly. Carrying a purse or shopping bag on the shoulder does not aggravate the hands and avoids putting pressure on the fingers that encourages ulnar deviation.

CHAPTER TWENTY-ONE

Corticosteroids

The anti-inflammatory effect of corticosteroids was an important discovery of modern medicine. Since their introduction in 1949, the use of cortisone (corticosteroids) in the management of rheumatic diseases has remained controversial. The potent effects corticosteroids have on joint inflammation like swelling, redness, warmth, and pain are well accepted, but come at a price. The price is side effects. The corticosteroids utilized in the treatment of arthritis are not the same as sex hormones in birth control pills or the anabolic steroids used in body building to increase muscle mass. In fact, cortisone breaks down muscle and so is catabolic, leading to weakness, muscle atrophy, and much more.

There are several different preparations of corticosteroids. Prednisone (Orazone) and methylprednisolone (Medrol) are two common oral preparations. They are relatively inexpensive. Corticosteroids are taken orally and by injection (parenteral). Corticosteroids are injected directly into swollen joints or an area of inflammation like bursitis, trigger points, or tendinitis for a more localized effect. Preparations for soft tissues include triamcinolone (Kenalog) or methylprednisolone (Depomedrol). Systemic effects from a single dose occur in all organ systems, regardless of the route of administration. Even localized injections have systemic effects. Injecting corticosteroid into one knee will result in some benefit to other joints. A localized corticosteroid injection transiently aggravates the control of diabetes because of its systemic effect on glucose control.

It has been reported that long term, low-dose oral prednisone (<10 milligrams/day) has been used in the treatment of approximately one-third of RA patients seen in clinical practice. Controversy exists as to whether there are benefits with regard to disease activity, functional capacity, or x-ray progression of the arthritis.

Side Effects of Corticosteroids

The major drawback of corticosteroids is serious side effects. Because steroids are frequently used in the treatment of arthritis, the delicate balance between efficacy and toxicity is monitored closely. If corticosteroids are used for prolonged periods, side effects do occur. Relatively low doses in a disease like RA (non-life-threatening illness) minimizes side effects as compared to the benefits. Many of the side effects are reversible and some are not. Unfortunately, weight gain is difficult to shed. A vertebral compression fracture secondary to corticosteroid-induced osteoporosis leads to a chronic painful back. Facial hair increases, but can improve. Menses may be missed. Patients on corticosteroids develop cataracts and glaucoma that continue. Corticosteroids aggravate hypertension and diabetes control, but improve as doses are discontinued. In large doses corticosteroids cause extreme anxiety, sleeplessness, and even psychoses that resolve as the dose is decreased. Capillary fragility and thin skin results in bruising easily, especially at the forearms. Almost any dose of corticosteroids creates an increased risk for infection. Corticosteroids are associated with an increase of gastritis or gastric ulcers.

Corticosteroids should not be avoided because of a concern for side effects. Doses should be kept to a minimum. Alternate day corticosteroids avoid some side effects, although some illnesses require daily dosing. If a medical problem is considered life-threatening or serious, high-dose corticosteroids (greater than 60 milligrams/daily) are required to achieve the therapeutic effect desired. In that situation, side effects occur until the dose is safely tapered.

Avascular Necrosis

A serious complication of corticosteroid use in rheumatic diseases is bone death (avascular/aseptic necrosis). The hip is often affected. The circulation to the femoral head of the hip is limited and when compromised, bone dies (necrosis). This results in collapse of the femoral head and disruption of the joint. Avascular necrosis can occur in multiple joints. Once there is collapse of the femoral head of the hip, treatment requires total hip replacement. Fat globules block the circulation and compromise blood flow. Increased lipids occur secondary to corticosteroids and contribute to the fat globules.

Adrenal Suppression

The adrenal glands produce cortisol (steroid). Cortisol maintains normal physiological functions of the body including blood pressure, fluids, and electrolyte balance of sodium and potassium. It is safe to take corticosteroids for periods of less than two weeks without significant suppression of the adrenal glands. Chronic use of corticosteroids results in suppression of the adrenal glands and the glands' ability to respond with extra steroid for emergencies or stress. After oral corticosteroids are taken for prolonged periods, it is best to taper slowly so that the adrenal glands resume production of steroid. While tapering corticosteroids, vigilance continues for reappearance of the signs and symptoms of the treated disease and evidence of adrenal insufficiency. Symptoms of adrenal insufficiency include fatigue and low blood pressure. Withdrawal symptoms of muscle, bone, and joint pain occur during the tapering of large corticosteroid doses.

During periods of extreme stress, the adrenal glands release large amounts of cortisol necessary to maintain physiological function in the normal individual. After prolonged oral corticosteroids, the suppressed adrenal glands do not release adequate quantities of cortisol to respond to stress quickly. During the perioperative period of surgery, adrenally suppressed individuals need supplemental intravenous corticosteroid doses to make up the difference of what the adrenal gland is not capable. Adrenal insufficiency continues as long as one year after discontinuing prolonged chronic oral corticosteroid usage.

Acutely, corticosteroids are given in multiple divided doses throughout the day, then eventually twice a day, with the larger dose in the morning and the smaller dose in the evening. All chronic corticosteroid users should carry identification describing their disease and steroid requirements.

Anti-inflammatory Effect

Because of their profound effect on inflammation, corticosteroids are the most potent anti-inflammatory agents known to man. The side effects associated with corticosteroids have been a motivating force behind research to find better and safer drug therapies in the treatment of arthritis. Other anti-inflammatories like NSAIDs do not contain corticosteroids. NSAIDs have a completely different benefit versus risk profile. The number of available NSAIDs has grown tremendously the last several years. If corticosteroids are given concurrently, NSAIDs can often be discontinued, avoiding added risk.

Many American citizens seek out relief for their arthritis at clinics south of the Mexican border. The medications prescribed at these clinics often include NSAIDs combined with corticosteroids. Although there is initial relief for some patients, many return home to find that the side effects of the corticosteroids are worse than the arthritis.

Initiation of Corticosteroids

Oral corticosteroids are started at any time during the course of RA or other forms of rheumatic illness. Corticosteroids provide enough relief until other drug therapies with fewer side effects become effective. There is no evidence that corticosteroids provide more than symptomatic relief in the treatment of arthritis. Corticosteroids bridge the gap and allow a breadwinner to continue to work. The decision to start oral corticosteroid therapy is an important one.

Some patients are never able to taper and discontinue corticosteroids. Long-term low-dose corticosteroids are required to suppress inflammation, regardless of alternative treatment programs in these individuals. Low-dose corticosteroids are defined by less than or equal to 10 milligrams of prednisone or an equivalent corticosteroid daily. In other serious rheumatic disease states like vasculitis or SLE, high-dose corticosteroid is required to suppress the immunologic responses. Once there is suppression, corticosteroids are safely tapered to lower levels. Corticosteroids disrupt the inflammatory cycle and allow a more normal state of health to return. Prednisone (40 milligrams/daily equivalent or more) defines high-dose steroids. Because both response and side effects of corticosteroids are dependent on dose size and the duration of treatment, it is crucial not to change doses without close monitoring. Every effort should be made to limit the use of corticosteroids to the shortest course of time. If maintenance treatment is necessary, the lowest possible corticosteroid dosage should be used.

Corticosteroid Side Effects
◊ increased appetite
◊ truncal obesity, moon facies
◊ hypertension
◊ capillary fragility (bruising)
◊ cataracts and glaucoma
◊ diabetes
◊ osteoporosis and fractures
◊ facial hair
◊ striae
◊ infections (shingles, thrush)
◊ peptic ulcer disease
◊ depression, mood changes
◊ anxiety, psychoses

CHAPTER TWENTY-TWO

Antirheumatic Drugs (DMARDs)

Drugs with the potential to reduce or prevent joint damage are disease-modifying antirheumatic drugs (DMARDs). Similar terms include second line or remittive agents. While NSAIDs and corticosteroids effectively alleviate symptoms, joint damage still occurs. DMARDs are the cornerstone of the treatment of RA and many other rheumatic illnesses.

Rheumatoid arthritis patients with active persistent synovitis, early onset, and poor prognostic indicators, despite adequate treatment, are candidates for DMARDs. Poor prognostic indicators include persistent fatigue and morning stiffness, persistent elevated markers of inflammation as evidenced by an ESR or CRP, persistent swelling and signs of inflammation of the joints, radiographic erosions, nodules, and a high titered rheumatoid factor or anti-CCP. These patients need early and aggressive treatment with DMARDs.

The decision to start a DMARD must be preceeded by a discussion with the patient, close relatives, or significant others about the risks versus benefits of the treatment and the expected outcome (informed consent). The best initial DMARD choice is not known; there are advantages to each. However, DMARDS do not play a role in the treatment of osteoarthritis, gout, fibromyalgia, or other non-inflammatory rheumatic illnesses.

Antimalarials

The relative cost, safety, and convenience of antimalarials make them an initial selection for patients with mild disease of RA or SLE. The beneficial effects of these drugs are determined after several weeks of therapy. The need for continuation of antimalarials is then decided. Antimalarials in combination with other DMARDs are common. Antimalarials were first used in the 1940s to treat malaria. Many years later, it was discovered that antimalarials were useful in the treatment of RA and SLE.

Antimalarials block ultraviolet light from damaging skin and have an anti-inflammatory effect. Interference with the immune response partly explains the beneficial effects. Unlike corticosteroids and immunosuppressive agents, they have no adverse effect on blood counts or an increased risk for infection. Individuals require only infrequent monitoring.

In SLE, antimalarials are effective in treating rash, arthritis, and serositis like pleuritis or pericarditis. Antimalarials are corticosteroid sparing. Patients on antimalarials requiring corticosteroids use smaller daily corticosteroid doses than those individuals who do not take antimalarials at the same time. Antimalarials improve constitutional symptoms like fatigue or malaise, but they do not have a role in the treatment of more serious manifestations of SLE, especially central nervous system and kidney disease.

In the treatment of RA, antimalarials are often added to existing DMARD therapy. In the future, antimalarials will be used less often as monotherapy in early RA because of the increasing effectiveness of new therapies.

The two most common oral preparations include hydroxychloroquine (Plaquenil) and chloroquine (Aralen). A third preparation, quinacrine (Atabrine) is not associated with retinal changes like hydroxychloroquine, but is associated with yellow pigmentation of the skin. Hydroxychloroquine is the only current antimalarial approved by the FDA and promoted specifically for RA. Chloroquine and quinacrine work more quickly and are more potent, but they are not as safe as hydroxychloroquine. Antimalarials cause some patients to experience headaches, muscle aches, and weakness. Stomach upset, loss of appetite, bloating, cramps, nausea, and vomiting occur but are infrequent and minor. Generally, antimalarial therapy is well tolerated. In psoriasis, there is concern that antimalarials aggravate the rash.

The side effect of most concern with antimalarials is changes of the retina. The changes are characteristic and dose-related on a daily basis. Hydroxychloroquine (400 milligrams/daily or less) is rarely associated with retinal disease. As with most medicines, greater doses are not necessarily better. If retinal changes are detected early and the medication discontinued, the changes of the retina reverse without loss of vision. Retinal examination is done once a year. Routine eye examination by an ophthalmologist including color vision and visual fields detect early changes that are more apt to be reversible. If the eye exam is scheduled within a few weeks of initiation of treatment, the medication is started before the eye exam. Antimalarials are slow-acting drugs. The beneficial effects in both RA and SLE occur over weeks. Only a small percentage of patients ever experience difficulty with antimalarials and most patients continue medicine.

Plaquenil is the most commonly prescribed antimalarial. The usual dose is 200 milligrams twice daily for many months. A missed dose will have no immediate effect on the disease course. Various dosing schedules are utilized. Just as the effects of antimalarials take weeks to occur, after discontinuation the benefits of antimalarials take weeks to disappear. Side effects have been reported to occur weeks after the medicine is discontinued.

Sulfasalazine

Sulfasalazine (Azulfidine, Azulfidine EN) is a drug that for many years has been used in the treatment of inflammatory bowel disease. Sulfasalazine has been available since the late 1940s. It seems to have both an anti-inflammatory and an antibiotic effect in the treatment of gastrointestinal disorders. Sulfa-allergic individuals should not take sulfasalazine.

Sulfasalazine is given early in RA or in combination with other remittive agents. Periodic blood monitoring is required. Although there are a number of serious side effects, most side effects are mild and readily reversible. Common side effects include headache, nausea, diarrhea, rash, and low blood counts. Men experience low sperm counts that are reversible upon discontinuation of the medicine.

The tendency has been to use sulfasalazine in refractory cases, but in these situations it works less well than other DMARDs. It is best to use it early in RA, when the response is inadequate to NSAIDs. It is used in conjunction with NSAIDs, corticosteroids, and other remittive agents. Sulfasalazine demonstrates clinical response after a relatively short treatment period. Sulfasalazine (500 milligrams) is given in divided doses. The maximum total dose is 3,000 milligrams/daily. Enteric-coated tablets (Azulfidine EN-Tabs) reduce stomach absorption and minimize gastrointestinal irritation and symptoms like nausea and vomiting. Like antimalarials, sulfasalazine will be used less often in early RA in the future because of the success of biologicals.

Methotrexate

Methotrexate (MTX) is the gold standard by which new DMARDs are evaluated and measured. It is the most frequent choice of initial DMARD. Approximately 60 percent of patients on MTX have a significant response, and it has the most predictable benefit of all available DMARDs; patients continue it longer than any other DMARD. The fact that MTX can induce cancers like lymphoma in a small number of RA patients remains a concern and requires a continued level of awareness.

Experts agree that one of the most meaningful advances in the treatment of RA over the past decade or more has been the acceptance and increasingly widespread use of MTX. First developed to treat cancer, MTX was approved by the FDA for the treatment of RA in 1988. Clinicians have widely accepted the use of MTX in the treatment of RA. Despite adverse effects, most patients tolerate MTX well. Patients improve rapidly in a few weeks, plateau at about six months, and then are maintained on treatment. Toxicities, rather than the lack of benefit, are the most common cause of discontinuing MTX. Fifty percent of patients will still be taking MTX five years after initiating the drug therapy.

Careful attention is directed toward adjusting dose levels of MTX therapy. Frequent individualized dose manipulations are necessary to continue the drug safely. It is likely that the initial oral dose of MTX will be changed because of a side effect. Toxicity increases with the dose. An appropriate initial starting dose for most patients is 7.5 milligrams weekly. The average dose is 15 milligrams weekly, but higher doses are used. Careful monitoring for toxicity is required during therapy. The weekly dose is taken either singularly or in divided doses over twenty-four hours.

Early experience with MTX discovered evidence of fibrosis of the liver. Unfortunately, abnormal liver function discovered on routine tests does not reflect structural changes of the liver. Patients who develop liver function abnormalities (liver enzyme elevations) that persist during treatment or after discontinuation of the drug require a liver biopsy. A liver biopsy is not recommended prior to therapy. Those patients already at an increased risk for liver disease, including alcoholics, should not take MTX. Alcohol consumption should be minimized or avoided. If any abnormalities of liver function occur, alcohol should be stopped and liver function tests reexamined. Regular monitoring of liver function tests is mandatory. Hepatitis C individuals should avoid MTX.

Other reported side effects of MTX include mild hair loss, low blood counts, nausea, and stomatitis. Occasionally, side effects require temporary discontinuance of therapy or lowering of the weekly dose. Folate is depleted while taking MTX and is responsible for some of the side effects. The concurrent use of folic acid (folate 1 milligram/daily) or multivitamins (folate 0.4 milligram/daily) minimizes some of the side effects and doesn't seem to interfere with the beneficial effects. Potentially dangerous lung inflammation induced by MTX is unusual, but is very serious.

Even when substantial anti-inflammatory effects are achieved from MTX, therapy exaggerates or induces rheumatoid nodules in some RA patients.

The reason for rheumatoid nodulosis is poorly understood and in some cases necessitates the discontinuation of MTX, surgery, or the addition of other drugs. Antimalarials or sulfasalazine help reduce the nodulosis occurring in MTX-treated patients.

Aspirin and other NSAIDs are used with MTX, but the potential for interaction exists. Corticosteroids are continued and gradually reduced once an MTX response is achieved. Concomitant use of other DMARDs has been studied and in some refractory MTX patients, combination DMARDs is effective. Anti-TNF drug therapy in combination with MTX is effective.

Once a response is achieved, MTX is reduced to the least effective dose. Improvement begins within three to six weeks in contrast to other DMARDs that take twelve to sixteen weeks to show response. Self-injectable doses of MTX have advantages over oral preparations. Injectable MTX is less expensive than oral tablets. After an injection, MTX goes to the tissues and bypasses the liver. The bypass effect exposes the liver to lower concentrations of the drug than oral preparations. If larger doses of MTX are necessary to control the arthritis, the initial bypass of the liver makes MTX safer. Injectable doses are similar to the oral doses.

Oral or injectable MTX is not associated with acute GI distress. Increased infection rates or the potential to induce lymphoma are related to the immuno-suppression that benefits the arthritis. Immunosuppression increases the risk of unusual infections (oral thrush, for example), and MTX should be avoided during concurrent infections or the flu. Since MTX causes birth defects, women of childbearing potential must use birth control. It is given to women with ectopic pregnancy to induce abortion. People with serious kidney or liver disease, alcoholics, or individuals with AIDS should not take MTX. It has no effect on fertility in women.

Azathioprine (Imuran) is a useful immunosuppressive drug for the treatment of rheumatoid arthritis. Azathioprine is used less frequently than MTX. Azathioprine is well tolerated, but initially requires frequent and close monitoring of the blood counts. Later, as the dose (100 to 200 milligrams daily) is stabilized the cell counts are done less often. The correct dose needed to suppress the disease is often judged by at least some suppression of the white cell count (leukopenia).

Gold Therapy

Intramuscular gold injections have been available for many years. Although rarely used now, gold injections deserve mention because of their significance. Weekly injections are required before beginning monthly maintenance therapy. Monitoring of blood and urine is required before each and every injection. Oral gold preparations like auranofin

(Ridaura) do not appear to be effective, cause diarrhea, and are rarely used. There are two available gold preparations given by intramuscular injection. These include oil-based gold aurothioglucose (Solganol), which is absorbed slowly from the muscle, and a faster absorbed preparation, gold sodium thiomalate (Aurolate). The fast absorption of gold is associated with lightheadedness as a result of hypotension (nitritoid reaction). The rapid absorption of gold sodium thiomalate dilates the blood vessels in a way similar to the effect of nitroglycerin. Nitritoid reactions do not occur with the slower acting preparation. For that reason, gold aurothioglucose is safer in older individuals who cannot afford the effects of hypotension. Initial gold injections include a small test dose to monitor for hypotension. Nitritoid reactions can occur any time during therapy.

Gold injections are given intramuscularly. Patients seldom complain about the injection, but rather about the required blood testing and frequent medical visits. Gold injections are cumbersome because of the patient's time commitment, monitoring, and potential side effects. Unfortunately, there is no test available to determine who will respond or develop side effects secondary to gold.

If the patient is medically supported and given adequate time, all side effects of gold therapy are reversible. Even so, many are serious, life threatening, and require that the gold be stopped immediately and never restarted. Dry, scaly, and itchy rashes are common and usually a nuisance. Rashes improve with lower doses of gold, delaying the frequency of injection, or applying topical steroid creams. Itching is relieved after taking antihistamines. Exfoliative skin reactions occur infrequently. Low blood counts occur commonly. Thrombocytopenia can be severe. Leukopenia increases the chance for infection and needs to be distinguished from Felty's Syndrome (RA, leukopenia, recurrent infections, and splenomegaly). Excess protein in the urine (nephrotic syndrome) is discovered early by monitoring with a urinary dipstick and usually reverses without harm to kidney function. Nephrotic syndrome will recover with time.

D-Penicillamine

Historically, D-penicillamine (Cuprimine, Depen) has been effective therapy. Dosing is convenient and requires a go-low and go-slow regime. Small doses (250 milligrams/daily) are initiated and increases are only made at about three-month intervals. More individuals will quit penicillamine than gold injections because of side effects, but just as many will respond, too. Penicillamine has many of the same side effects as gold, including a lupus syndrome. Loss of taste may occur. Pencillamine is given to penicillin-allergic individuals. The popularity of other DMARDs has decreased the use of penicillamine.

Penicillamine is slow acting over many months. Daily doses are taken on an empty stomach two hours before or after meals. The medication is taken daily in divided doses. Few patients respond to very low doses (250 milligrams/daily). The maximum daily dose is 1,500 milligrams.

Cyclosporine

Cyclosporine (Sandimmune, Neoral) is an immunomodulating agent approved for the treatment of RA. Cyclosporine has made organ transplantation possible. It is a drug that has significant effects on the immune system. Cyclosporine's long-term efficacy and toxicity in RA remains unclear. Disadvantages include costs relative to other second-line agents and potential kidney toxicity. During organ transplantation of the heart, liver, or kidney the immunologic benefits of cyclosporine justify its indefinite use, even if some kidney dysfunction occurs. In contrast to organ transplantation, the dose used for the treatment of autoimmune disease is lower. However, some patients with RA require prolonged treatment, and kidney toxicity is of concern. Cyclosporine should not be given to individuals with any preexisting kidney disease or hypertension. Since both the disease and drug therapy impact kidney function, kidney function is monitored closely. Evaluations include the monitoring of blood pressure, blood, and urine. If kidney function worsens compared to baseline, the dose must be reduced. Kidney toxicity is manageable, but not negligible. NSAIDs work in concert and depress kidney function. Withdrawal of NSAIDs is not always feasible. Other side effects include facial hair growth, acne, diarrhea, nausea and vomiting, and swelling of the gums.

Whether DMARDs should be given sequentially or additively for patients remains controversial. More than ever before, the trend is to use DMARDs in combination. In many patients with severe RA partially responding to MTX, clinical improvement is noted with the addition of cyclosporine compared to MTX alone.

The rationale for the use of cyclosporine depends on the role of T cell function and cellular immunity as compared to B-cell function and humeral immunity. In RA, there is abundant evidence for the role of T cells in the inflammatory process. On the other hand, in SLE, humeral immunity is more important than cellular immunity. There is less rationale for the use of cyclosporine in SLE.

Cyclosporine appears to reduce inflammation, reduce pain, and improve mobility. In kidney transplant patients, cyclosporine is associated with an increased frequency of cancer. It generally takes between four and eight weeks for symptomatic relief.

Liquid cyclosporine is more palatable than soft gelatin capsules (25 milligrams, 100 milligrams). Doses are given twice daily. The dose is dependent upon weight. For the average individual, low doses range between 150 and 200 milligrams/daily. At low doses, side effects are mostly reversible. Since it can alter the absorption of the medication, grapefruit juice should be avoided within an hour of the medication.

Leflunomide

Leflunomide (Arava) was the first in a number of new RA therapies approved after a prolonged period of time without any new drug therapies for RA. Leflunomide works by blocking the overproduction of immune cells that are responsible for the inflammation caused by arthritis. Early studies have shown just about as much improvement as MTX in comparison to placebo. Radiographic progression of RA is slowed by the administration of oral leflunomide.

Side effects include diarrhea, rash, hair loss, and liver toxicity. Diarrhea occurs in as many as one third of the patients. Hair loss reverses if the drug is stopped. Regular monitoring is required. Elevation of the liver enzymes signals problems and the need for discontinuation. After consumer groups requested the FDA to withdraw leflunomide from the market because of associated liver failure, the FDA decided the benefits to RA patients outweighed the risks and did not withdraw the drug. The concur-

rent administration of MTX increases the potential for liver problems and must be used cautiously. After initiating leflunomide, potential toxicity typically occurs soon.

Women must not get pregnant on leflunomide. Animal studies suggest leflunomide causes numerous birth defects. Effective birth control is required. Most drugs rapidly clear from the body after the last dose is taken, but leflunomide lingers for months. Women who wish to become pregnant after taking leflunomide take cholestyramine to remove leflunomide before conception. To minimize any risk of birth defects, men wishing to father a child should discontinue the use of leflunomide and also take cholestyramine. If leflunomide must be stopped, the manufacturer has devised an elimination procedure. A full eleven-day course of cholestyramine medication is followed by two separate laboratory blood tests at least fourteen days apart to insure a very low drug level. If the drug levels are too high, a repeated drug elimination procedure is necessary. After the drug elimination procedure, the risk of having a baby with birth defects is low and should be no higher than the risk in the general population. Without the elimination procedure, it could take up to two years to reach a low blood level of leflunomide.

Because blood levels increase slowly, the first three days of oral leflunomide is given as a loading dose (100 milligrams/daily) rather than the usual dose

(20 milligrams/daily). If side effects are suspected, the dose can be reduced to a 10-milligram oral tablet/daily. Leflunomide does not require dose increases, although lower doses are used if tolerability is a problem. The drug is taken without regard to meals, concomitant NSAIDs, or corticosteroids. The loading dose or larger daily dose is associated with diarrhea is some individuals.

A positive effect is evident by one month, stabilized by three to six months, and then maintenance doses continue. Radiographic studies demonstrate a slowing of disease progression.

Biological Agents

Research has shown that tumor necrosis factor (TNF) plays a central role in RA. TNF appears to stimulate inflammatory cells and drive the inflammation of arthritis. TNF is a cytokine or chemical mediator in the joint fluid of both normal joints and those with inflammatory arthritis. Since 1998, the FDA has approved anti-TNF agents for the treatment of RA. Currently available TNF inhibitors for the treatment of RA include etanercept, infliximab, and adalimumab. Infliximab is approved for use only in combination with methotrexate and is administered at four- to eight-week intervals after an initial loading regime. Etanercept and adalimumab are self-administered subcutaneous injections approved for use as monotherapy or in combination with MTX.

There have been few studies comparing anti-TNF treatments with other active DMARDs.

Etanercept

Etanercept (Enbrel) is a genetically engineered protein produced by recombinant DNA technology. Etanercept binds specifically to tumor necrosis factor (TNF) and blocks its action. TNF is a natural occurring cytokine that promotes inflammatory and immune responses. TNF plays a critical role in the inflammatory processes of RA and the resulting joint damage. Elevated levels of TNF are found in the joint fluid of RA patients. Etanercept is given as a self-injection subcutaneously once or twice a week. Responses appear within weeks after initiation of therapy and nearly always by three months. After discontinuation, symptoms return. Etanercept is approved for those RA patients with symptoms of moderate to severe disease who have had an inadequate response to one or more DMARDs. Etanercept is used in conjunction with MTX or alone as monotherapy. Allergic reactions to etanercept are rare, although itching or rash at the injection site occurs. Experience with etanercept for several years has been mostly uneventful. Treatment is discontinued in patients with serious infections. Live polio, smallpox, and intranasal influenza virus (Flumist) vaccines are avoided in patients receiving anti-TNF agents. Other side effects occur infrequently, but include headache, nasal congestion, dizziness, sore throat, cough, generalized weakness, abdominal pain, rash, lung problems, shortness of breath, or inflammation of the sinuses. Etanercept is also approved for psoriatic arthritis, psoriasis, juvenile arthritis, and ankylosing spondylitis.

Infliximab

Infliximab (Remicade) neutralizes the biological activity of tumor necrosis factor. This monoclonal antibody works quickly. RA patients feel substantially better within weeks of the first intravenous infusion. Studies have confirmed that relief continues for months. Infliximab is diluted in sterile water and given with saline as an intravenous infusion over two hours. After the initial dose, infusions are repeated at two weeks, six weeks, and then every eight weeks. Occasional patients require greater doses or a more frequent infusion schedule. Methotrexate is given concurrently to suppress neutralizing antibodies against infliximab. Neutralizing antibodies contribute to the need for increasingly larger and more frequent dosing of infliximab (Remicade creep). Infliximab is effective treatment and provides relief for most patients for the entire eight weeks between treatments. The most common side effects include upper respiratory infections, headache, nausea, coughing, and diarrhea. Very few people stop the treatment because of side effects.

Some people notice mild reactions during the infusions like itching, chills, low back pain, difficulty breathing, or low blood pressure. When reactions occur, they resolve quickly if the infusion is stopped or the infusion rate slowed. The rate of the infusion often correlates to infusion reactions, so that if the intravenous rate is kept slow, fewer reactions occur. Subsequent infusion reactions necessitate premedicating with acetaminophen, antihistamines, or even corticosteroids. Following infusions, the patient resumes a normal schedule.

Infliximab is also approved for use in Crohn's disease, ulcerative colitis, ankylosing spondylitis, and psoriatic arthritis.

Adalimumab

The third anti-TNF drug therapy available for the treatment of RA is adalimumab (Humira). It has a prolonged effect compared to some of the other anti-TNF drug therapies. A subcutaneous self-injection of adalimumab is given every two weeks. Traveling with anti-TNF medication becomes difficult because of the necessity of keeping the medicine refrigerated. There is some suggestion that this genetically engineered protein is more human-like than other drug therapies and will be less associated with allergic responses. The yearly expense of all anti-TNF medication is relatively similar and expensive. Adalimumab is also approved for psoriatic arthritis.

Anakinra

Anakinra (Kineret) is an alternative to other biological agents. Anakinra inhibits a different natural cytokine protein (IL-1) of the immune system than TNF. Interleukin-1 plays a role in the inflammation of arthritis. Anakinra is an interleukin 1 receptor antagonist (IL-1 RA). Daily self-injections cause injection site reactions the first few weeks that resolve slowly during the continuation of therapy. Inhibition of the cytokine interleukin 1 is not as effective in RA as inhibition of the cytokine tumor necrosis factor. Anakinra may be more effective in other rheumatic illnesses where interleukin 1 plays an important role. Anakinra does not have as significant association with increased infections as other biological agents. Currently the only approved indication is in the treatment of rheumatoid arthritis.

Abatacept

Abatacept (Orencia) is a biological agent indicated for moderate to severe rheumatoid arthritis patients who have not been helped by other DMARD therapy. Abatacept is a selective co-stimulatory modulator and prevents the activation of T-lymphocytes implicated in the inflammation and damage of rheumatoid arthritis. When T cells are activated or turned "on" they start a chain of events that lead to the inflammation, pain, and damage occurring in rheumatoid arthritis. This is different from the other biologics, which work at the cytokine level of the immune system process. Cytokines are the proteins that appear after a T cell has already been activated and drive the inflammation process of RA—often leading to joint damage and destruction. Most other biological agents block the important cytokine TNF. Since abatacept affects the immune system in rheumatoid arthritis differently than the anti-TNF agents, it may be useful in those individuals failing to achieve a therapeutic effect with anti-TNF agents.

Like all medicines that affect the immune system, abatacept can cause side effects, which can include serious infections, allergic reactions, and malignancies. The more common side effects with ORENCIA are headache, upper respiratory infection, sore throat, and nausea.

In a study of patients who had not responded well enough to MTX alone, patients given abatacept plus MTX or MTX alone at twelve months did better with combination therapy. The patients who received abatacept plus MTX had progression scores that were about 50 percent lower than those who received MTX alone.

Abatacept may be used as monotherapy or concomitantly with DMARDs other than anti-TNF agents. The dose is based on weight and given intravenously over thirty minutes on a monthly basis.

Rituximab

Rituximab (Rituxan) was the first monoclonal antibody approved for the treatment of cancer. Rituxan continues to be used successfully in non-Hodgkin's lymphoma. Years later, research has resulted in an indication for the treatment of rheumatoid arthritis in combination with methotrexate. Rituxan targets specific immune system CD20 B cells (lymphocytes) and can improve the symptoms and signs of RA through six months. Rituxan is administered differently than the other biological therapies. Rituxan therapy requires two separate intravenous infusions over several hours on different days separated by two weeks. To avoid infusion reactions the patients are often premedicated with acetaminophen and corticosteroid. The infusions are given slowly over a few hours. Rituximab is an important addition to the drug therapy of rheumatoid arthritis, but its exact role remains to be determined. Although rituximab has some unique side effects during the treatment of lymphoma, they do not appear to be significant in the rheumatoid arthritis patients. However, infections continue to be a concern.

Caution about Biologicals

All biologicals and concomitant immunosuppressive therapy alter the immune response, including the response to infection. Those individuals with chronic infections or a history of recurring infection should avoid these agents. Diabetics with poorly controlled blood sugars are at increased risk for infections and should avoid biologicals.

All patients anticipating the start of biological therapy should be screened for evidence of latent tuberculosis with a skin test or chest x-ray. The skin test should be read at forty-eight to seventy-two hours and is considered positive in individuals who have greater than or equal to 5 millimeters of induration (firmness, not erythema). After active TB has been excluded, a minimum of nine months of anti-TB therapy is instituted for those individuals with a positive skin test never before treated. Anti-TNF therapy can be started within a month of the anti-TB therapy. Anti-TB therapy includes oral isoniazid (INH) along with pyridoxine (B6 vitamin).

There is a concern about the induction of cancer with anti-TNF agents, especially lymphoma. Clinically, this is not a major obstacle. Regardless of therapy, lymphomas are more frequent in RA patients, but still unusual. RA patients have at least a twofold increased risk for lymphoma compared with the general population. Since the release of anti-TNF therapies, surveillance has associated these agents with central nervous system disease like multiple sclerosis. In patients with multiple sclerosis, anti-TNF agents are avoided. Early studies investigating anti-TNF therapies in heart failure were halted after it was clear that there was no benefit. Some heart patients in these studies did worse. Anti-TNF medications are not given to patients with heart failure.

The observation that the lack of efficacy with one anti-TNF therapy does not preclude benefit with another anti-TNF suggests that the immune effects of these drug therapies differ in a given individual. Since there are three commercially available anti-TNF medications, research is needed to identify the characteristics that predict a response to different anti-TNF therapies. Newer biological agents appear to be effective in the treatment of RA in some patients failing the anti-TNF therapies.

Prosorba Column

The prosorba column is a medical device approved for patients with moderate to severe RA who have not experienced significant relief from MTX or at least two other DMARDs. The device is the size of a soup can and filters immune complexes from the blood. The idea is to remove antigen antibody complexes responsible for the effects of RA. The procedure is done weekly for twelve weeks. Each session lasts about two hours. Blood is drawn from the patient and separated into cellular components and plasma. The plasma with the immune complexes is passed through the column. Antibodies selectively stick to the column and are removed. The cleansed plasma is returned to the patient. Almost one-half

of the treated patients in clinical studies achieved improvement for twenty to seventy-five weeks. Improvement occurs within three to four months after the initiation of treatment. If necessary, the cycle is repeated. The projected cost and time commitment for this procedure makes it an undesirable option for some people.

Tetracyclines

Trials have demonstrated the efficacy of tetracycline (minocycline) in improving the clinical parameters of RA. One trial showed long-term benefit of minocycline and a decrease in radiographic progression in a subset of patients. Further research is necessary to define the exact role of tetracyclines in the treatment of RA as a DMARD. Currently, tetracyclines are infrequently used DMARDs. Dizziness is the most commonly observed side effect. As with other tetracyclines, minocycline is potentially injurious to the liver.

Future Drug Therapy

Research for new drugs in the treatment of RA and other rheumatic illnesses is keen. New drugs show promise in blocking the biological processes that perpetuate joint inflammation and destruction of joints. Several drugs that block cytokines or other mediators of inflammation are under investigation. In the normal immune system, cytokines are thought to regulate pro-inflammatory activity and contribute to the inflammatory state of arthritis.

Other biologicals in the research pipeline target other cytokines or the receptors on the cell surface they trigger. Almost all show some efficacy. New drug therapies for RA have prompted some rheumatologists to suggest, "This may be the best time to get rheumatoid arthritis, since the treatment is so effective and can slow the progression of the arthritis." Excitement is tempered with concern for the incidence of infection and cancer with these therapies.

Goals of Treatment

The goal of treatment with DMARDs is to begin early and prevent joint damage. The diagnosis of and type of arthritis must be certain. On occasion this is difficult and the natural course of the disease must be observed. Few conditions other than inflammatory arthritis are appropriate to treat with remittive agents, although their usefulness is expanding in other rheumatic conditions.

All DMARDs are slow in acting. There is no test to determine who will respond or react. The results of a clinical drug trial do not always correlate to the results for a single individual with rheumatoid arthritis. Efficacy is determined on an individualized basis, and each and every patient must be monitored carefully for side effects. Each DMARD is unique. The choice of DMARD depends on the need for convenience, the requirements for monitoring, the cost of medications, the time until expected benefit, the frequency of side effects, other medications, complicating medical problems, previous experience of the patient and physician, the ability to comply, and finally, the manifestations of the arthritis.

CHAPTER TWENTY-THREE

NSAIDs

NSAIDs are the most commonly prescribed class of drugs. They are used in all forms of arthritis and minor pain. More than 70 million prescriptions for NSAIDs are written annually in the United States. Seventeen million Americans take NSAIDs on a regular basis. Over 10 percent of the population greater than sixty-five years of age use NSAIDs.

Traditional NSAIDs include ibuprofen (Motrin, Advil, Nuprin, Medipren), naproxen (Naprosyn, Aleve, Naprelan), sulindac (Clinoril), diclofenac (Voltaren, Voltaren XR), piroxicam (Feldene), ketoprofen (Orudis, Oruvail), diflunisal (Dolobid), nabumetone (Relafen), etodolac (Lodine, Lodine XL), oxaprozim (Daypro), indomethacin (Indocin, Indocin SR), and others. In low doses, many NSAIDs are available at the drugstore over-the-counter. Aspirin and salicylates are traditional anti-inflammatories because of their similar effects.

Types of Nonsteroidal Anti-inflammatories
◊ traditional anti-inflammatories
◊ COX-2 selective agents

NSAIDs are the foundation of drug treatment for inflammatory arthritis. The FDA approves a large number of NSAIDs for arthritis. Most NSAIDs inhibit mediators of inflammation (prostaglandins). Preventing the formation of prostaglandins lessens the pain and inflammation of arthritis. Although most NSAIDs work in the same fashion, there are differences between their efficacy and tolerability.

COX-2 selective NSAIDs (coxibs) appear to have fewer GI side effects, no effect on platelets, and fewer bleeding problems than traditional NSAIDs. Coxibs selectively inhibit the prostaglandins generated by the COX-2 isomer of cyclooxygenase. Preserving the other COX-1 dependent prostaglandins maintains important protective mechanisms of the body and minimizes side effects, especially gastric ulcers and bleeding. Celecoxib (Celebrex) is the only available COX-2 selective drug. Rofecoxib (Vioxx) and valdecoxib (Bextra) were withdrawn after several years of successful use because of side effects. Other coxibs are still under investigation.

Side Effects of NSAIDs

The benefits and side effects of NSAIDs vary among patients. Someone taking the same drug for the same reason may not experience the same adverse events of others. Likewise, one person may not experience benefits experienced by the next. Occasionally, drugs lose their effectiveness, even though the same drug was efficacious earlier. Manufacturers of NSAIDs have pursued different indications for their drugs with the FDA to make their products unique. Among NSAIDs, some differences in the chemistry do exist, but there is limited information on the practical consequences of such differences.

Many available traditional NSAIDs are now generic.

Traditional NSAIDs have equivalent side effects as salicylates or aspirin. NSAID side effects are more common in elderly patients. Adverse effects include peptic ulcer disease, renal failure, congestive heart failure, bleeding, hypertension, central nervous system (CNS) toxicity, and more. Central nervous system effects include poor memory, fatigue, reduced concentration, depression, and headache. NSAID therapy should be avoided in patients with a history of gastrointestinal or kidney disease and monitored more carefully in the elderly. NSAIDs are apt to increase systolic blood pressure. Patients over fifty years of age are more apt to have systolic hypertension. The blood pressure is monitored during NSAID use in all patients. Less common side effects of NSAIDs are skin rashes, abnormal liver function tests, asthma, headache, and neck stiffness that resembles meningitis. The majority of NSAID-related side effects are reversible once the drug is stopped. During continued use, regular blood counts, hepatic enzymes, and kidney function are monitored every few months. Combinations of NSAIDs increase the chance of side effects.

Salicylates are NSAIDs. Non-acetylated salicylates (Disalcid, Trilisate) minimize the side effects of acetylated salicylates (aspirin), since they have no effect on platelets and do not prolong the bleeding time. Aspirin and other salicylates decrease platelet stickiness. Traditional NSAIDs have the same effect on platelets as aspirin. Even small doses of aspirin affect platelets and bleeding times for weeks. Cardiac patients take one baby aspirin (81 milligrams/daily) for its anticoagulant effect. Full anti-inflammatory doses of aspirin are easily measured in the blood. Aspirin blood levels approaching toxicity cause tinnitus, yet some individuals tolerate even higher doses of daily aspirin.

Peptic Ulcer Disease and NSAIDs

Traditional NSAIDs increase the incidence of peptic ulcer disease and gastritis. Inflammation of the gastric mucosa results in ulcerations or erosions that perforate the stomach wall and cause bleeding. NSAID gastropathy describes gastritis and peptic ulcers occurring as a result of NSAIDs. Upper GI endoscopy is necessary to biopsy the gastric mucosa and determine evidence of infection or cancer. Only a small percentage of traditional NSAID users ever develop serious complications of ulcer disease. It is estimated that more than 15,000 deaths occurred annually secondary to NSAIDs prior to the development of coxibs. NSAID complications make the development of safer NSAIDs increasingly more important. Coxibs are safer than traditional NSAIDs on the GI tract. Unfortunately, analysis of clinical drug trials with coxibs reveals an increased risk for heart attack and

stroke. There is a suggestion that even traditional NSAIDs carry the same cardiovascular risk. The FDA has called for a black box warning about this risk for all NSAIDs.

H2 receptor antagonists help heal gastric ulcers and are taken concurrently with anti-inflammatories. H2 receptor antagonists include cimetidine (Tagamet), ranitidine hydrochloride (Zantac), famotidine (Pepcid), and nizatidine (Axid). Proton pump inhibitors are more potent acid-blocking medications, prevent ulcer disease, and include rabeprazole (Aciphex), pantoprazole (Protonix), omeprazole (Prilosec), lansoprazole (Prevacid), and esomeprazole (Nexium). Sulcrafate (Carafate) topically heals gastric ulcers and has no systemic effect. H2 receptors and proton pump inhibitors prevent or decrease the production of stomach acid. Many are available over-the-counter in small doses. There is concern that preventing acid formation will mask GI symptoms and put patients at an increased risk for GI bleeding.

Misoprostol (Cytotec) is a synthetic prostaglandin analog that has the ability to put prostaglandins back into the stomach wall. Prostaglandins protect the stomach from its own acid production. Acid production is not altered. Misoprostol causes diarrhea and uterine cramping, and must be avoided in women of childbearing potential because of its effects on the uterus. The concurrent use of misoprostol with NSAIDs (Arthrotec) decreases the chance of developing gastric ulcers.

Various delivery modes are used to avoid GI distress because of anti-inflammatories, including enteric coatings or time-released preparations. Ecotrin (aspirin) is enteric-coated. Enteric coatings prevent the breakdown of NSAIDs in the stomach and allow the release of the medication farther down the GI tract. Since the adverse effect of NSAIDs is systemic and results in the depletion of gastric wall prostaglandins, the beneficial effects of enteric coatings are minimal. Food provides similar and minimal benefit.

Additional risk factors for peptic ulcer disease and its complications include smoking, alcohol, and the concurrent use of corticosteroids and anticoagulants. Peptic ulcer disease can be asymptomatic. There may be no history of nausea, vomiting, or diarrhea. Even gastrointestinal bleeding occurs frequently without any early symptoms.

NSAIDs Are Symptomatic Therapy

NSAIDs are often utilized in the treatment of musculoskeletal pain and inflammation and are well tolerated. They are used in conjunction with other medications in the treatment of more serious rheumatic illness, but do not have the ability to suppress the immune system (immunosuppressive). NSAIDs are symptomatic treatment only. Anti-inflammatories do not change the course of arthritis. In low doses, NSAIDs are used for their analgesic properties and not their anti-inflammatory effects. In low doses, NSAIDs are available over-the-counter at the pharmacy without the need for a prescription.

Aspirin

There are many different preparations of aspirin. Buffered aspirin is surrounded with an antacid. Enteric-coated aspirin is encased in a shell, which passes intact through the stomach to dissolve in the intestine. Sustained-release aspirin (Zorprin) releases aspirin over several hours. Full anti-inflammatory doses of aspirin include twelve or more tablets (325 milligrams/tablet) of regular aspirin daily. Toxic aspirin levels cause tinnitus, yet elderly individuals do not hear the ringing. If ringing occurs, decreasing the daily aspirin dose by one tablet a day will drop blood levels and the tinnitus resolves. The range between the toxic and therapeutic levels is narrow.

Aspirin has been used for many years for arthritis. Considering Americans take millions of tablets daily, aspirin is one of the safest medicines available.

Aspirin, like NSAIDs, blocks the production of prostaglandins. The full effects of aspirin take several days until a therapeutic level is achieved. Besides aspirin's anti-inflammatory effects, aspirin has analgesic effects and lowers temperature effectively.

Aspirin Side Effects

Aspirin irritates the stomach lining and causes heartburn, indigestion, nausea, vomiting, and even bleeding, just like traditional NSAIDs. Non-acetylated aspirin causes fewer problems than regular aspirin. Allergic reactions occur rarely. Individuals with aspirin allergy and nasal polyps aggravate their asthma when they take aspirin.

Aspirin inhibits platelet aggregation. Aspirin's antiplatelet effect lasts the lifetime of a platelet and causes bleeding in susceptible people. Patients with peptic ulcer disease should never use aspirin. Gastrointestinal bleeding could be catastrophic. The antiplatelet effect of aspirin makes it useful in those individuals threatened by stroke or heart attack. One daily baby aspirin (81 milligrams/tablet) is rarely associated with problems, but is highly effective for anticoagulation. The advantages of aspirin far outweigh the risks in these individuals. Aspirin should be avoided prior to surgery, since it can increase the risk of unnecessary bleeding.

It is important to read the labels of over-the-counter medications that contain aspirin. While aspirin is a wonder drug with a long and interesting history, it can be harmful and should only be taken as part of a treatment program of arthritis. Alcohol should be avoided while taking aspirin, since alcohol can also irritate the stomach. Alcohol and aspirin together are double trouble.

COX-2 Agents

Postmarketing studies of COX-2 selective inhibitors reveal a trend towards increased heart attacks and strokes in patients compared to placebo or comparative drugs. Studies released during late 2004 reported new information about patients with coxibs and risk for heart attacks. A study of rofecoxib (Vioxx) showed significant increase in cardiovascular risk after eighteen months as compared to placebo and resulted in the withdrawal of the drug by the pharmaceutical manufacturer.

Investigational studies of valdecoxib (Bextra) in the high-risk coronary artery bypass graft (CABG) setting reveals higher rates of serious cardiovascular events in those patients receiving high doses of valdecoxib compared to placebo. Serious skin reactions have been reported in patients using valdecoxib. Some of these reactions resulted in death. The seriousness of these reports resulted in an FDA request and then voluntary withdrawal of valdecoxib in 2005.

Though celecoxib (Celebrex) has never been tested for cardiac safety, many experts believe it poses the same cardiac risk as rofecoxib. Unfortunately, with the cloud of suspicion hanging over the entire COX-2 class, the FDA is likely to demand a higher order of safety before it approves further members of this class of drugs. For this reason, the next generation of COX-2 drugs in development like etoricoxib (Arcoxia) and

Public Health Advisory by the FDA about NSAIDs
◊ The FDA requested that valdecoxib (Bextra) be voluntarily withdrawn from the market due to an unfavorable risk versus benefit profile of the drug.
◊ The FDA asked all manufacturers of marketed prescription NSAIDs revise their prescribing information to include a black boxed warning, highlighting the potential for increased risk of cardiovascular (CV) events and serious gastrointestinal (GI) risks. This is the most severe warning the FDA can place on a product's label.
◊ A medication guide will be required to be distributed with every NSAID prescription.
◊ The product labeling for non-prescription or over-the-counter NSAIDs will be revised to include more specific information about potential CV and GI risks, as well as skin reactions.

Alternatives to COX-2 Anti-inflammatory Agents	
Pain Relief	Acetaminophen (Tylenol), tramadol (Ultram), and non-aspirin salsalates (Disalcid or Trilisate)
Relief for Inflammation	Traditional anti-inflammatories like ibuprofen (Advil, Motrin, Aleve, and others)
Topical Agents	Rubs, gels OTC, lidocaine patches, capsaicin cream

lumiracoxib (Prexige) are delayed. Subsequent to all this controversy about the COX-2 medications, the FDA issued a Public Health Advisory during April 2005.

While investigating coxibs in usual doses and naproxen versus placebo, another study reported new information. There was no significant increase in cardiovascular risk for patients on coxibs compared to placebo; however, there was an apparent increase in risk for patients on naproxen compared to placebo. This was surprising information, since naproxen is not a COX-2 selective agent and has been available for many years. The last few years, naproxen (Aleve) has been available without prescription. This information has led to a black box warning on all NSAIDs of potential risks for heart.

CHAPTER TWENTY-FOUR

Immunosuppressive Drug Therapy

Immunosuppressive agents are effective in the treatment of systemic lupus erythematosis or other autoimmune disease. The suppression of the immune system reduces disease activity in major organs like the kidney (nephritis) and is used in addition to or instead of corticosteroids. Immunosuppression is corticosteroid sparing and helps avoid the side effects of corticosteroid therapy. Although immunosuppressive drugs have serious side effects, close monitoring avoids trouble. Immunosuppressive drug therapy provides significant benefit and prolongs life in serious rheumatic disease.

Immunosuppressive Agents Commonly Used
◊   azathioprine (Imuran)
◊   cyclophosphamide (Cytoxan)
◊   methotrexate (Rheumatrex, Trexall)
◊   mycophenolate (Cellcept)

Mechanism of Action of Cytotoxic Therapy

Rapidly dividing cells are most susceptible to the effects of immunosuppressive drugs. Azathioprine (Imuran) and cyclophosphamide (Cytoxan) are utilized in autoimmune diseases. Other cytotoxic drugs include chlorambucil (Leukeran), nitrogen mustard (Mustargen), mycophenolate (Cellcept), and methotrexate (Rheumatrex,

Trexall). Immunosuppressive drugs target rapidly dividing cells like primary malignant cells, antibody-producing cells of the immune system, blood cells, hair cells, and reproductive cells like the ovaries and testes. In autoimmune disease, immunosuppressive drug therapies suppress the hyperactive cells of the immune system.

Side Effects of Cytotoxic Therapy

Side effects with cytotoxic drug therapies occur as a consequence of oversuppression of the immune system. Oversuppression reduces the cellular components of the bloodstream including the red cells (anemia), white cells (leukopenia), or platelets (thrombocytopenia). Anemia adds to fatigue. Leukopenia increases the risk for infection and decreases the ability to fight infections. Thrombocytopenia results in excess bleeding. Oversuppression of hair cells results in baldness. The cytotoxic affects on the reproductive cells results in difficulty conceiving or even sterility.

During immunosuppressive drug therapies, regular blood samples are monitored. At the initiation of therapy or change of dosing, samples are checked more often. Suppression of the total white count is a measure of the correct azathioprine dose. In most cases, azathioprine is well tolerated. Experience with kidney transplant patients suggests there might be a slightly increased risk

for cancer in those patients taking higher doses for prolonged periods of time.

Cyclophosphamide is the most important immunosuppressive in the treatment of vasculitis. Potential side effects include increased risk for cancer, cystitis, infection like shingles, hair loss, and temporary or permanent sterility. Cyclophosphamide is given orally or intravenously.

Dosing of Cytotoxic Therapy

Serial monthly intravenous boluses of cyclophosphamide are given for lupus nephritis. This therapy is well tolerated and especially important in SLE patients with nephritis. Oral doses of either azathioprine or cyclophosphamide on a daily basis require periodic monitoring of the blood cell counts. The two drugs are never taken at the same time. Azathioprine is not given intravenously.

Mycophenolate (Cellcept) is used with success in several autoimmune illnesses. Treatments with cyclophosphamide are associated with serious related problems including hair loss, infertility, blood disorders, and even bladder cancer. The most common side effect of mycophenolate is gastrointestinal complaints and low white blood cell counts. The reduction of dosage will almost always resolve the symptoms.

Immunosuppressive agents are not given indefinitely. Although these drugs are the standard of practice in many autoimmune and rheumatic illnesses, the prescribing physician must provide an informed consent to the patient. An informed consent includes a thorough discussion of the risks and benefits of such medicine.

CHAPTER TWENTY-FIVE

Biological Drug Therapy

Biological drug therapy neutralizes cytokine proteins responsible for the inflammation of arthritis. The effects are quick and profound.

Approved Biological Agents
◊   Enbrel (etanercept)
◊   Remicade (infliximab)
◊   Humira (adalimumab)
◊   Kineret (anakinra)
◊   Orencia (abatacept)
◊   Rituxin (rituximab)

Etanercept

Etanercept (Enbrel) is a protein produced by recombinant DNA technology. Etanercept binds specifically to tumor necrosis factor (TNF) and blocks its action. Tumor necrosis factor is a naturally occurring chemical in the body that promotes the inflammatory and immune responses. It plays an important role in the inflammatory processes of RA and the resulting joint damage. Elevated levels of TNF are found in the joint fluid of RA patients. Etanercept is a subcutaneous self-injection given once or twice a week. Once-a-week injections (50 milligrams) are supplied in prefilled syringes. Twice-a-week injections (25 milligrams) require dilution and mixing of drug. Responses appear within two weeks after initiation of therapy and nearly always by three months. After discontinuation of medicine, the symptoms of arthritis return. Etanercept is recommended for those RA patients with symptoms of moderate to severe disease, who have had an inadequate response to one or more DMARDs. Etanercept is used in conjunction with more recognized therapies like MTX, but also as mono-therapy. Allergic reactions to etanercept are rare. Itching or rash at the injection site occurs. The long-term effects of anti-TNF medications are not known, especially with the body's defense mechanisms against infection or malignancies. Patients who develop a new infection while undergoing treatment with etanercept are monitored closely. Treatment is discontinued in patients with serious infections. Other side effects occur infrequently, but include headache, nasal congestion, dizziness, sore throat, cough, weakness, abdominal pain, rash, shortness of breath, or inflammation of the sinuses. Early reports demonstrated exacerbations of multiple sclerosis.

Infliximab

Infliximab is a monoclonal antibody that specifically targets tumor necrosis factor. Infliximab effectively relieves the signs and symptoms of RA. Infliximab works quickly, and a patient with RA feels substantially better within weeks of the first therapy. In studies of long duration, continued treatment with infliximab provided long-lasting relief, while the medication was continued. Infliximab is given concurrently with MTX.

Infliximab is diluted in sterile water and given as an intravenous infusion with saline. The infusion is given slowly over two hours. The dose is calculated based on weight. After the initial dose, infliximab is repeated at two weeks, six weeks, and then every eight weeks or six times a year. It is effective treatment and provides relief for the entire eight weeks between treatments.

The treatment is well tolerated. Mild reactions like itching, chills, difficulty breathing, or low blood pressure occur during the infusion. When reactions occur, they resolve if the treatment is stopped or the rate of infusion slowed. Subsequent infusion reactions require premedicating with acetaminophen, antihistamines, or even corticosteroids. The most common side effects include upper respiratory infections, headache, nausea, coughing, and diarrhea. Very few people stop the treatment because of side effects.

Neutralizing antibodies to infliximab develop in a small portion of patients. It is possible that these neutralizing antibodies accelerate the clearance of infliximab and explain infusion reactions or shorter duration of response. Concomitant MTX treatment reduces the incidence of neutralizing antibody formation. Antinuclear antibodies occur after anti-TNF therapy in some patients, but less often when MTX is given concurrently. The incidence of more specific antibodies for the disease systemic lupus erythematosis is unusual.

Adalimumab

Adalimumab (Humira) is a monocloncal antibody that strongly binds to human anti-TNF. Adalimumab is self-injected subcutaneously from a prefilled syringe every two weeks. The clinical response improves with the addition of MTX, yet adalimumab is also given as monotherapy. Minor itching or redness is common after the self-injections of adalimumab. Allergic reactions like hives occur occasionally, but serious allergic reactions are most unusual. The efficacy is comparable to the other anti-TNF agents.

Guidelines in Heart Failure for All Anti-TNFs

Researchers know that TNF levels are elevated in heart failure and associated with decreased strength of the heart's contraction. Early heart failure studies with anti-TNF therapy were encouraging, but later studies lacked evidence for benefit and in some cases showed increased death rates. Since the release of anti-TNF agents, postmarketing studies report further cases of new or worsening heart failure. This has led to a warning of the use of these medications with known heart failure patients.

Currently, specialists recommend the following guidelines for all available anti-TNF medications in the treatment of RA and heart failure.

Guidelines in Heart Failure and Anti-TNF Therapy

◊ Screen patients for heart failure.
◊ Monitor patients with compensated mild heart failure closely.
◊ Stop anti-TNF agents in all patients with new onset heart failure.
◊ Avoid anti-TNF therapy in patients with moderate to severe heart failure.

Guidelines with Past/Active Infections for All Anti-TNFs

Serious bacterial infections, tuberculosis, or fungal infections have occurred with all the anti-TNF agents. Most cases of TB in those patients taking anti-TNF agents occur as a result of reactivation of previous TB. Screening procedures like skin testing and chest x-ray decrease the incidence of reports of TB associated with anti-TNF drug therapy. Investigators have learned that TNF plays a role in the normal response to TB.

All TNF blocking agents and concomitant immunosuppressive therapy alter the immune response, including the response to infection. Those individuals with chronic infections or a history of recurring infection should avoid anti-TNF treatment. Therapy should not be started in patients with active infection and discontinued if serious infection occurs while on therapy. All patients are given yearly flu vaccines and pneumonia (Pneumovax) vaccines every five years prophylactically.

Guidelines Regarding Infections and Anti-TNF Drug Therapy

◊ Screen for past TB with a skin test (PPD) or chest x-ray.
◊ Individuals with a positive PPD should be treated with anti-TB therapy.
◊ Avoid treatment in patients with recurrent past bacterial infection.
◊ Take appropriate vaccinations.
◊ Stop treatment during active infections.

Guidelines in Cancer for All Anti-TNFs

The incidence of lymphoma is increased among people with RA and increases with the severity of the arthritis. All anti-TNF agents have been associated with the occurrence of lymphoma. A definite cause and effect relationship between lymphoma and anti-TNF ther-

apy remains possible. No specific guidelines exist for previous cancer patients.

Guidelines about Cancer and Anti-TNF Therapy

◊ Incidence of lymphoma is increased in RA.
◊ Incidence of lymphoma is increased with anti-TNFs.
◊ Effects on previous cancers with anti-TNFs are unknown.
◊ Increased vigilance for all potential side effects is required.

Anti-TNF agents appear to be among the most effective treatments available for RA. The response is generally rapid, often occurring within a few weeks. Not all patients have a clinical response. Some individuals respond to one anti-TNF agent and not another. It is useful to try a second anti-TNF agent, if there is no clinical response to the first. Anti-TNF therapy is avoided in patients with multiple sclerosis or heart failure, and given carefully to diabetics. Since abnormal blood tests occur infrequently, monitoring is rarely needed.

Anakinra

Interleukin-1 is a chemical mediator of the immune system. A natural inhibitor controls the action of interleukin-1. In RA, levels of the natural inhibitor are low. Animal models with low inhibitors of interleukin-1 develop an inflammatory arthritis like RA. The approval of anakinra (Kineret) an antagonist to interleukin-1 provides an alternative biological agent to the anti-TNF medications. A daily self-injection is required because of the short duration of the drug once administered. Clinical responses are good, but not as effective as anti-TNF therapies. Like the other biologicals, response improves with the addition of MTX. Common adverse experiences are injection site reactions occurring in most individuals. The skin reactions are red, swollen, and itchy. The skin reactions resolve after a few weeks of continued therapy. Serious infections are of concern as with the other biologicals. Periodic blood monitoring is recommended because of occasional low blood counts.

CHAPTER TWENTY-SIX

Other Treatments

Topical Agents

An exciting concept in pain management is the use of transdermal medications placed directly on the skin. Topical creams avoid side effects of oral medications. Unlike oral medications, topical agents are designed to provide a high concentration of drug locally without significant absorption into the blood. Topically applied NSAIDs, such as ketoprofen gel, penetrate the skin and provide concentrations of the anti-inflammatory to a targeted area. Formulated gels readily penetrate the skin. The skin acts as a drug reservoir and releases medication slowly. The transdermal route is effective for many medications. Using the right combination of oral and topical medications controls pain with less reliance on narcotics. Unfortunately, compounding pharmacies are the only locations with the ingredients and expertise to formulate the combinations necessary for topical gels or creams. Topical pain compounds have not been extensively studied to verify their effectiveness.

Topical creams, oils, gels, ointments, and sprays from the drugstore are applied directly to the tender areas of the skin. The natural impulse to gently rub areas of soreness of a painful joint or muscle brings comforting warmth into the area. Home remedies have been used for years as rubs for the same reasons. Rubs contain analgesics and other ingredients that are well absorbed into the skin. The massaging effect while applying creams has a benefit all of its own. There is a potent placebo effect. The most common active ingredients include salicylates. Menthol, oil of wintergreen, camphor, and eucalyptus oil irritate the skin. Irritants stimulate the nerve endings and cause sensations masking pain.

Capsaicin

Capsaicin is found in chili peppers. Capsaicin creams rubbed over the joints reduce pain sensation by blocking the ability of the nerve endings around a joint to send pain impulses to the brain. Capsaicin creams are applied in small amounts directly on the skin over areas of pain several times daily. Capsaicin cream (Zostrix) comes in low-dose (0.035 percent) or high-dose (0.075 percent) concentrations. The pain will return once the cream is no longer applied. It can take a few weeks for the capsaicin to work. Initially, it may be associated with a burning sensation that resolves with time. Capsaicin is useful for the pain of herpes zoster (shingles). Capsaicin cream will irritate the eyes if it gets into the mucous membranes.

Joint Injections

Intra-articular corticosteroid injected into a swollen painful joint is effective and well tolerated. Results are variable and last for several days to months. Commonly used corticosteroids include triamcinolone hexacetonide (Aristospan), triamcinolone diacetate (Aristocort), and betamethasone (Celestone). Corticosteroid preparations are insoluble and minimize systemic effects. Even so, an injection of corticosteroid into one knee will usually help the other knee. The same joint

should not be injected too often. As a rule of thumb, it is not recommended to inject several large joints at any one setting. Intra-articular corticosteroid is not injected into a suspected septic joint. Only a few compounds are safely injected within the joint. Antibiotics, anesthetics (1 percent Lidocaine), and radiographic dye are safely placed within the joint space. Anesthetic benefits are usually short-lived.

Arthrocentesis

Aspiration of fluid from a tensely swollen space provides immediate comfort. Swelling stretches pain fibers and nerves. If there is no other intervention to disrupt the inflammatory cycle, the fluid reaccumulates quickly. Analysis of the fluid identifies infection or other cause of swelling. Fluid examined under a polarizing microscope can identify crystals of urate (gout) or calcium pyrophosphate (pseudogout). Monosodium urate crystals are negatively birefringent and calcium pyrophosphate crystals (CPPD) faintly positively birefringent. Joint fluid white cell counts differentiate inflammatory (RA) or non-inflammatory (OA) arthritis. Gram stains, glucose levels, and cultures document evidence of sepsis.

Viscosupplementation

Intra-articular injections of hyluronan or hyaluronic acid (HA) are indicated for the treatment of the pain of OA of the knee in patients who have failed to respond adequately to conservative other measures such as NSAIDs or acetaminophen. There are five available preparations including hyaluronate (Hyalgan, Euflexxa, or Supartz), hyan G-F 20 (Synvisc), and hyaluronan (Orthovisc). Hyalgan and Supartz are all natural, while Synvisc has been altered. Orthovisc is ultra-pure and natural. All the preparations are given as a minimum of three weekly injections over two weeks. Hyaluronic acid is a natural viscoelastic agent found in normal joint fluid. For many years, veterinarians have known of hyaluronic acid's beneficial effect in animals because of its cushioning and lubricating properties. Joint fluid functions as a lubricant and shock absorber because of its hyaluronic acid content. As a consequence of OA, the joint accumulates extra fluid, while hyaluronic acid levels diminish. The joint fluid loses its normal elasticity, viscosity properties, and its ability to act as a shock absorber. Injections of hyaluronans restore the elastic and viscous nature of the fluid, lubricate the joint, and allow the fluid to absorb the painful shocking motion of walking or running. Pain is relieved for six months. Injections are useful in those individuals intolerant of therapies like NSAIDs or trying to delay surgery. Studies have shown that viscosupplementation reduces the symptoms of OA of the knee about as effectively as NSAIDs. In the future, it is likely hyaluronans will be injected into other OA joints.

Viscosupplementation Agents
◊ Hyalgan
◊ Synvisc
◊ Euflexxa
◊ Orthovisc
◊ Supartz

If beneficial, the series of hyaluronans injections is repeated after six months. The side effects of hyaluronans are mild and primarily related to the risks of the injection. Unique to Synvisc injections are pseudoseptic post-injection flares that mimic infection. The day following the injection the joint rapidly swells and is associated with intense pain. The acute inflammatory response requires immediate joint fluid aspiration to examine for the possibility of infection. Intra-articular corticosteroid and oral anti-inflammatory agents provide immediate relief. The fluid is sterile and not septic. Pseudoseptic reactions are not associated with the natural hyaluronan preparations. Repeat injections of Synvisc following a pseudoseptic reaction are not appropriate.

Fish Oils

Fish oils lessen the inflammation of arthritis and its symptoms. Fish oils contain omege-3-fatty acids that reduce the production of arachidonic acid. The breakdown products of arachidonic acid are mediators of inflammation. Arachidonic acid is formed from fatty acids in a normal diet, but omega-3-fatty acids in fish oil are different. The fish oils taken in a normal diet prevent the formation of arachidonic acid and inhibit painful inflammation. Studies have proven that omega-3-fatty acids have this effect, but the benefits are small. Initial studies utilized large quantities of fish oils, much more than what any normal diet contains. Cod liver oil contains small amounts of the fatty acids found in fish oil supplement, but huge amounts are still necessary to match the quantities used in research studies.

Copper Bracelets

Many arthritis clinics are established on the basis of unproven remedies. Promoters of unproven remedies abound and tend to make exaggerated claims. There is no proven remedy that will cure arthritis, be effective in all forms of arthritis, or is beneficial just because it is natural. Most unproven remedies are expensive and somewhat unusual. Testimonials are limited and not proof of validity. Other unproven remedies include copper bracelets, horse liniment (DMSO), sitting in uranium mines, magnets, and special diets.

Glucosamine and Chondroitin Sulfates

Laboratory studies reveal that glucosamine stimulates production of cartilage-building proteins. Chondroitin inhibits cartilage-destroying enzymes and is anti-inflammatory. Glucosamine and chondroitin are marketed as dietary supplements and promoted to benefit patients with OA. There is no compelling evidence that one is better than the other. Studies done on these substances do not meet the stringent requirements of a well-conducted clinical trial. These criteria include sufficient numbers of similar patients, under similar circumstances, in a double-blinded fashion, over a sufficient duration of time, and by reputable investigators. So far, these substances appear to be more of a marketing success than treatment for any form of arthritis.

Glucosamine is commercially derived from the shells of shrimp, lobsters, and crab. Chondroitin is obtained from cow cartilage. There is no dietary source of glucosamine. It is only available as a nutritional supplement. The basic mechanism of action remains unknown.

Glucosamine and chondroitin are readily available at health food stores and are not regulated by the FDA. A combination of glucosamine hydrochloride and low molecular weight chondroitin sulfate (Cosamin DS) is heavily advertised to revitalize stressed cartilage cells, maximize cartilage production, provide pain relief, and improve joint health. The minimum oral dosage is 1,500 milligrams daily in divided doses. Studies reveal that glucosamine is not always the same concentration from brand to brand or even bottle to bottle of the same brand. Characterizing glucosamine as a cure without additional proof of results from testing is irresponsible. It is important that people who take these supplements do not stop taking their conventional therapies. At best, glucosamine is comparable to a modest anti-inflammatory, but without the ability to rebuild cartilage or modify the joint. It takes a few months to produce any significant improvement with these supplements.

Most reported complaints with these supplements are mild in nature and predominately affecting the gastrointestinal system. Almost all complaints are reversible upon stopping the supplement. No study has found any serious side effects from either glucosamine or chondroitin. The most common side effects are increased intestinal gas and softened stools. People with diabetes monitor their blood-sugar level carefully when using these supplements. There have been no reports of allergic reactions. Since glucosamine is made from shellfish, people allergic to seafood should use it cautiously and watch for reactions. As for chondroitin, it can cause bleeding in people who have a bleeding disorder.

The Glucosamine/Chondroitin Ar-thritis Intervention Trial (GAIT) initiated by the National Institutes of Health was a large study that included almost 1600 patients with painful knee osteoarthritis. Patients were randomly assigned to receive glucosamine hydrochloride, sodium chondroitin sulfate, a combination of both supplements, celecoxib, or placebo. The study clearly showed no benefit in patients with mild-to-moderate knee OA, but a preselected subgroup of patients with moderate-to-severe knee OA did benefit from the combined supplements. Adverse events in the GAIT study were mild. Unfortunately, the results of this study were still not clear enough to recommend these supplements to all patients.

Herbal Supplements

Consumers spend more than $12 billion on natural supplements each year and sales continue to grow. Herbal supplement sales have more than doubled in the past decade. Users proclaim herbal remedies are natural and make them feel better. They also claim to have fewer side effects than other available medications. Even so-called functional foods contain some herbal remedies to perk you up and others to calm you down. Fashionable soda drinks now contain herbal supplements. Americans make more visits to nontraditional physicians than to their family doctors.

The rapid expansion of herbal medicines comes at some risk for the American consumer. None of these products are regulated as well as over-the-counter medications or foods. Deregulation of the herbal industry allows manufacturers to make product claims on labels without first getting them approved by the Food and Drug Administration (FDA). Prior to deregulation, lengthy clinical trials had to be completed that were time-consuming and expensive. The FDA requires that herbal supplements list all plants and chemicals on the label. When you open the bottle of a nutritional supplement, you really do not know what's in it.

The groundswell of American interest in herbal remedies is curious, since herbs have been widely used in Asian cultures for thousands of years. Even modern Europe has a long tradition of accepting herbal remedies. By contrast, the United States has lagged behind. Today, at least part of the aging population of America has become disenchanted with Western medicine and seeks out more control over their health. Herbal medicine may be just what the doctor ordered.

Giant pharmaceutical companies are also becoming involved. At least some of this popularity is motivated by consumer demand for different ways to maintain health. Conventional medicine is often perceived as cold and remote or synthetic as compared to the natural substances of herbal preparations. Of course, the active ingredient of an herb is a chemical. If the doctor is inacces-

sible, the clerk at the health food store is not. A rediscovery of the healing powers of plants only marks a return to an ancient form of medicine still used by the majority of the world's population. Many current modern medicines are derived from herbs, including aspirin from white willow bark.

CHAPTER TWENTY-SEVEN

Menopause

Menopause affects a woman's response to her arthritis and other treatments. All postmenopausal women experiencing vasomotor symptoms should consider estrogen replacement therapy (ERT). Estrogen is usually taken alone, but in some patients combined with progestin. Estrogen replacement therapy relieves many of the symptoms associated with menopause, including hot flashes and vaginal dryness. It provides protection against coronary heart disease and osteoporosis. Coronary heart disease is the leading cause of death among postmenopausal women and osteoporosis is the most common cause for fracture. Estrogen therapy decreases the risk for hip fracture by about 25 percent.

Side Effects of Estrogen Replacement Therapy (ERT)

Women who take unopposed estrogen for years are at risk for developing endometrial cancer. Combination therapy with a progestin and estrogen eliminates the risk for cancer in women who have an intact uterus. Women who take estrogen for many years are also at risk for developing breast cancer, stroke, or heart disease. The degree of risk remains controversial. Other side effects such as bloating, breast tenderness, headache, or irritability are mild. While taking hormones, menstrual spotting raises concern for endometrial cancer and the need for endometrial biopsy.

The decision to take ERT is a complex one. In those women who have had a hysterectomy and require ERT, there is no reason to add a progestin. If an individual is at an increased risk for breast cancer, the risk of hormonal therapy outweighs any benefits. In women with no particular risk factors for cancer and who do not have a uterus, treatment with estrogen alone is acceptable. The Women's Health Initiative raised concern for increased heart attack and stroke besides cancer for any women taking ERT. For this reason, many women are no longer taking any ERT.

Designer Hormones

An alternative to traditional hormones for postmenopausal women is raloxifene (Evista). Raloxifene is a selective estrogen receptor modulator (SERM) and activates specific estrogen receptors, while it does not activate others. Raloxifene has estrogen-like effects on bone and increases bone mineral density, but to a lesser extent than estrogen and, on lipid, decreases metabolism. Most important, raloxifene lacks estrogen-like effects on breast and uterine tissue. Without that effect, it does not cause breast tenderness or vaginal bleeding, does not increase the risk of breast or uterine cancer, and does not require concomitant progesterone treatment if a women still has her uterus.

Side effects of the therapy include blood clotting, hot flashes, and leg cramps. SERMs do not treat the vasomotor symptoms of menopause. New SERMs are expected in the near future. Menopause signals the beginning of a new phase in a woman's life, a time when risk for osteoporosis begins to increase dramatically.

Soy as Hormone Replacement

The concern about increased risk with ERT has left millions of women scrambling for an alternative. Soy protein containing estrogen-like compounds (isoflavones) is suggested for an alternative. It appears from studies that a daily dose of soy has no effect on bone loss, cholesterol levels, or mental function in postmenopausal women over sixty years of age as was initially suggested by early studies.

CHAPTER TWENTY-EIGHT

Clinical Drug Trials

Clinical drug trials provide opportunities to try new medications for the treatment of arthritis. There is no magical pill or cure for the treatment of arthritis. Neither is there any special drug, herbal medicine, surgery, dietary supplement, or other therapy that is clearly more advantageous than all the rest. Joint replacement has been the most important advancement in the treatment of arthritis during the past many decades, but drug therapy still offers the chance to prevent the destruction of joints before the need for surgery or joint replacement. Physician experts like rheumatologists favor drug therapy, with the judicious use of other interventions interspersed among them. Other interventions include hydrotherapy, stress reduction, and even acupuncture for pain control. There are several reasons for the utilization of medications. Historically medications work, at least to some degree, and drugs make sense with the current degree of our knowledge and understanding of the disease processes in arthritis. Most current research for new medicines is done in the United States by pharmaceutical companies. The United States is the leader of drug research. Together these companies continue to invest billions of dollars a year, more than the entire federal budget for the National Institutes of Health, the American premier health research institute. Of all the drugs approved by the FDA from 1981 to 1990, over 90 percent were discovered by pharmaceutical industry scientists, less than 10 percent at universities in the United States and other labs, and only 1 percent at government labs.

The Wealth of Medical Information

The pharmaceutical companies have obvious reasons for making such commitments. The challenges of finding a cure or relief for chronic diseases are greater than ever before; so are the scientific knowledge and technical resources at our disposal.

The wealth of information about disease process doubles every few years.

There is a huge market and need for new medicine, both in the U.S. and the world. Patients and families insist that we continue to explore new medicines to find cures that will make a difference for those individuals that have developed one of the more than one hundred different forms of arthritis. New science has opened up bits of information and knowledge never previously understood. We have more opportunities than ever before to treat diseases differently. Rather than just understanding the consequence of arthritis, we now have a better understanding of the mechanisms of disease at a cellular level and even within the cell or intracellular level. We have knowledge now that we did not understand just a few years ago.

America has been more successful than any other country in providing the right mix of incentives to keep research moving forward. Nearly one-half of the world-class drugs introduced over the past two decades came from the laboratories of American companies. No other country even came close. In other words, drug research is big business driven by the needs of patients, researchers, scientists, and investors. The financial expense of this research has been tremendous, but the rewards will be even greater.

Preclinical Testing

The pharmaceutical companies have established large laboratories and research teams throughout the world. New super-computing and technologies enable them to screen hundreds of compounds and to patent them immediately. Based on the knowledge of disease, drugs can now be designed and built molecule by molecule to interact at a cellular level specific for a disease state. This process takes considerable time and expense. Initial testing is confined to the laboratory and test tube. Eventually, it must be tried in living animal experiments. This preclinical testing will characterize the effects of the drugs on models of the disease. There has been criticism of animal experimentation, yet it enables researchers to predict at least some of the effects in humans. A major difficulty is finding animal models that mimic human disease. Results are very different in animals than humans. If testing is successful, the pharmaceutical company then asks the FDA for permission for further experimentation. The preclinical results are submitted and reviewed first by the FDA. At that time, the company requests an Investigational New Drug Application Approval (INDA) to begin testing in humans. If the FDA is satisfied with the review and decides that the potential benefits of testing in humans outweighs the risks involved, the stage is set for clinical trials.

The Institutional Review Board

All clinical drug trials must be approved by an Institutional Review Board (IRB). The boards review the ethics and appropriateness of human experimentation. There are many of these at hospitals, universities, or other areas around the country. They exist to protect the patient during human experimentation and consist of a cross section of individuals including scientists, medical doctors, pharmacists, nurses, clergy, and other people from the community. Essentially, the IRB reviews the study protocol, the patient's informed consent, the investigator and site, and the progress of the study to determine that the risks are reasonable in relation to the potential benefits. These built-in safeguards are designed to protect patients and their rights, and to prevent misleading promises or outcomes.

Phases of Clinical Trials

Clinical trials of experimental drugs in humans are done in three phases. Each successive phase involves a larger number of volunteer subjects. Even after a drug is released clinical trials continue. Clinical drug trials are double-blinded. Neither the patient nor the doctor knows who is receiving the new medicine or the placebo.

The Challenge

Pharmaceutical research is a complex and challenging process. It may be met with failure at any stage. Of the thousands of compounds synthesized annually at major pharmaceutical companies, only a few will make it to a developmental stage, and of these, only a few will make it through a process that can take as much as a decade and cost an average of $800 million for each new drug that emerges from a company's pipeline. As with other inventions and discoveries, new chemical compounds with the potential to become medicines are protected by patent laws that grant inventors exclusive rights. After the patent expires, the invention passes to the public domain, the world of generic medicines. U.S. patent rights are traditionally granted for seventeen years from the date of grant. Additional research eventually shortens the remaining useful life of a patent to six or seven years once a new drug reaches the marketplace. It is during this time that the pharmaceutical company must recover the enormous expense of research and development. Occasionally, unusual circumstances or changes of the drug will allow an extension of time of the exclusive rights. The longer period of exclusivity for a specific drug by a particular pharmaceutical company the greater chance they have of recouping their costs and making a profit for their shareholders. Once a drug falls into the realm of generics, the retail costs usually come down and the profit margins diminish.

Clinical trials are usually conducted in, but not limited to, large metropoli-

---

Phases of Clinical Drug Trials

◊ **Phase I Clinical Trials** focus primarily on safety, and gather preliminary data on the effectiveness of a new compound. A wide range of doses of the compound are usually administered to a small group of healthy volunteers under close supervision. This is often in a hospital or in a rigidly controlled setting.

◊ **Phase II Clinical Trials** last longer and focus on the compound's safety and effectiveness against the illness it was orginally designed to treat. Strict guidelines for informed consent are observed so that the potential benefits and risks are clearly explained to the patients. Some of the patients will receive a placebo. Placebos are sugar pills that have no active ingredients.

◊ **Phase III Clinical Trials** are the final stage. Researchers confirm the results of earlier tests in large geographical patient populations.This takes several years and includes up to several thousand patients. Large geographically diverse groups are sought to eliminate the effects of possible unique genetic characteristics of patient populations, or local events that could alter drug response or monitoring, for example an outbreak of hepatitis in one community.

◊ **Phase IV Clinical Trials** occur after FDA approval of the medication. Even after the drug has received FDA approval after the New Drug Application (NDA) process, companies will continue to conduct post-marketing studies to monitor safety issues.

---

tan areas or university centers. However, private clinicians often contribute significantly to such research. Recruitment can sometimes be difficult at a university. Private physicians have access to large number of patients with established disease. Patient populations in large teaching institutions have already often participated in clinical trials. Physicians-in-training often lack the experience necessary to do studies, do not have access to many patients, and do not have the advantage of following the same patient during the length of the study.

Volunteers

Only patients who wish to participate in a clinical drug trial should. It should be entirely voluntary and treatment should not be based just on willingness to participate. A volunteer is permitted to quit the study at any time, although in fairness to the study and its success at the time of initiation of the study, a well-informed volunteer should be committed to finish the study as long as they know the benefits and risks. Even after signing an informed consent a patient can leave the trial at any time and receive other conventional medical care without penalty. The informed consent must be read and signed before any study-related procedure or other action occurs. In addition, the investigator should explain the informed consent in detail and answer any and all questions the volunteer asks. An informed consent should leave the volunteer with an understanding of the protocol including the number of visits and procedures, previous studies with the medicine to date and known side effects, and other alternative, standard, or recognized treatments available. The informed consent must be written in language easily understood by the patient.

Patients in clinical drug trials are among the first to receive the benefits of new research before it is widely available to others. However, just as the effects of standard treatments can't be entirely predicted, neither can the results of an experimental treatment.

Participants in clinical drug trials are monitored closely according to the strict guidelines of the protocol. Their participation becomes part of a larger project carried out in many areas and by many investigators who can then pool their ideas and results. It is hoped then that the knowledge gained is shared to the benefit of all patients with the same illness.

To determine the appropriateness of entering a clinical drug trial, a patient has a number of issues to consider. Some illnesses cause symptoms and even death unrelated to treatment. Therefore, unavoidable risks of the disease must be weighed against the benefits and risks of the new research treatment. Even standard treatments cannot predict guaranteed results or the absence of side effects. The demands of some studies can be significant for some patients who already do not feel well, although the new therapy has the potential to help. If a patient receives a placebo, there may be no benefit at all and the disease worsens with precious time lost. For some individuals with limited resources, clinical trials provide an opportunity to access health care or a specialist knowledgeable of their illness, and provide opportunities for further care or directions after the study.

The myths and fears of clinical drug studies and human experimentation can be frightening. Some individuals will think of themselves as "guinea pigs in the laboratory." These ideas result from the fear of the unknown. It is imperative that the patient understand the informed consent and that anxieties are eased. During a research study, monitoring and observation is meticulous. It is believed that study patients actually receive better care than patients receiving conventional care. If, during a study, it is clear that the treatment being received is not in the best interests of the patient, the patient should be discontinued from the study.

Recent events with newly released drug therapies have led to the belief that all clinical trial results should be published and reviewed by peers, whether the results are positive or not. It is hoped that this will then lead to a better understanding of the drug therapy, disease, and future safety to patients.

Resources

Arthritis Foundation

1330 West Peachtree Street
P.O. Box 1900
Atlanta, GA 30326
Phone: (800) 283-7800 (toll free)
Internet: http://www.arthritis.org

American College of Rheumatology

1800 Century Place, Suite 250
Atlanta, GA 30345
Phone: (404) 633-3777
Internet: http://www.rheumatology.org

American Physical Therapy Association

1111 North Fairfax Street
Alexandria, VA 22314-1488
Phone: (703) 684-2782
Phone: (800) 999-2782, X3395 (toll free)
Internet: http://www.apta.org

American Academy of Orthopedic Surgeons

P.O. Box 2058
Des Plains, IL 60017
Phone: (800) 824-BONE (toll free)
Internet: http://www.aaos.org

Centers for Disease Control and Prevention

1600 Clifton Road
Atlanta, GA 30333
Phone: (800) 311-3435 (toll free)
Internet: http://www.cdc.gov

Food and Drug Administration

5600 Fishers Lane
Rockville, MD 20857
Phone: (301) 443-3170
Internet: http://www.fda.gov

Lupus Foundation of America, Inc. (LFA)

2000 L Street, N.W., Suite 710
Washington, DC 20036
Phone: (202) 349-1155
Phone: (800) 558-0121 (toll free)
Fax: (202) 349-1156
E-mail: lupusinfo@lupus.org
Internet: http://www.lupus.org

National Fibromyalgia Association

2200 N. Glassell Street, Suite A
Orange, CA 92865

Phone: (714) 921-0150
Fax: (714) 921-6920
Internet: http://www.fmaware.org

National Institute of Arthritis and Musculoskeletal and Skin Diseases (NIAMS) National Institutes of Health

1 AMS Circle
Bethesda, MD 20892-3675
Phone: (301) 495-4484 or
(877) 22-NIAMS (toll free)
Phone: (301) 565-2966
Fax: (301) 718-6366
E-mail: NIAMSInfo@mail.nih.gov
Internet: http://www.niams.nih.gov

National Osteoporosis Foundation

1150 17th Street N.W., Suite 500
Washington, D.C.
20036-4603
Phone: (202) 223-2226
Internet: http://www.nof.org

National Sjogren's Syndrome Association

5815 N. Black Canyon,
Suite 103
Phoenix, AZ 85015-2200
Phone: (602) 433-9844
(800) 396-NSSA (toll free)
Internet: http://www.sjogrens.org/

National Psoriasis Foundation

6600 SW 92nd Avenue
Suite 300
Portland, OR 97223
Phone: (503) 244-7404
Phone: (800) 723-9166 (toll free)
Fax: (503) 245-0626
Internet: http://www.psoriasis.org/home

National Center for Complementary and Alternative Medicine

P.O. Box 7923
Gaithersburg, MD 20898-7923
Phone: (301) 519-3153
Phone: (888) 644-6226 (toll free)
Internet: http://www.nccam.nih.gov

The Paget Foundation

120 Wall Street, Suite 1602
New York, NY 10005-4001
Phone: (212) 509-5335
Fax: (212) 509-8429
E-mail: pagetfdn@aol.com
Internet: http://www.paget.org

Scleroderma Foundation

89 Newbury Street STE 201
Danvers, MA 01923
Phone: (800) 722-HOPE
Phone: (978) 750-4499
Fax: (978) 750-9902

E-mail: SFinfo@scleroderma.org
Internet: http://www.scleroderma.org

Spondylitis Association of America

14827 Ventura Blvd. Suite 222
Sherman Oaks, CA 91403
Phone: (800) 777-8189
Internet: http://www.spondylitis.gov

Index

for measuring bone mineral density
(BMD), 23
of osteoarthritis (OA), 9, 74
quantitative computerized tomography
(QCT), 24
of rheumatoid arthritis (RA), 9

Z

Zoloft, 48

About the Author

Malin Prupas, MD is a board-certified rheumatologist with over twenty-five years of experience caring for patients with many forms of arthritis and related conditions. His current responsibilities include acting as the medical director of the Arthritis Center of Reno. Dr. Prupas is an associate clinical professor of medicine at the University of Nevada School of Medicine and is board certified in both rheumatology and internal medicine. He is a consultant for several major pharmaceutical companies and has conducted multiple clinical drug trials.

Dr. Prupas has been a principal investigator of more than 250 different clinical drug trials of investigative medicines for the treatment of arthritis and related conditions. He has worked with all the major pharmaceutical companies including Amgen, Pfizer, Merck, Centacor, Lilly, Immunex, Wyeth, Beringer Ingleheim, Endo, Abbott, Tap, and many others. Several of these drugs are currently available and have been approved by the Food and Drug Administration.

Dr. Prupas was a member of the charter class of the school of medicine at the University of Nevada, Reno. He transferred to Tufts University School of Medicine, Boston, and received his MD degree in 1975. The completion of his internal medicine training followed in Southern California. He completed a fellowship in rheumatology and immunology at USC-LA County Medical Center in 1980 before he relocated with his family to Reno, Nevada. Dr. Prupas is a Fellow of the American College of Physicians and the American College of Rheumatology.